"The paradigm has shifted and tl
The days of trying to build up sh
als and inserts are being replace
approach – barefoot running. Asl   ....,
this is the ideal way to build foot stability, balance, and prevent
injury."

Michael Fredericson, M.D.
Professor, Department of Orthopaedics & Sports Medicine
Head Team Physician, Stanford Track & Field
Stanford University School of Medicine

"Every question answered on running barefoot with a mix of true
stories of everyday runners and science to back them up. The
book was informative, well referenced, and an enjoyable, easy
read."

Marc Silberman, M.D.
NJ Sports Medicine and Performance Center

"I enjoyed this carefully researched book. It has some excellent
and practical information that I had not seen in *Born to Run* or
magazine articles on barefoot running."

Mike McGehee
Princeton University Cycling Team 1990-1994
Associate Professor of Material Science and Engineering,
Stanford University

"This book will make you question the science behind your
running shoes. With humor and insight, Mukharji addresses the
benefits of barefoot running while focusing his attention on the
concerns and hesitations that most of us have about casting our
shoes aside. His interviews with other barefoot runners open us
up to a world without running shoes, and his tips and techniques
make the reality of barefoot running ours for the taking."

Amy Eastwood, Ph.D.
University of Virginia Track Team, 1998-2002

"What goes on your feet should be a conscious decision - a decision informed by this thoroughly researched and well-argued book."

Alexander Gagnon, Ph.D.
Long time runner
Member of Team USA ITU International Aquathlon 2005

"Whether you run in shoes or barefoot, the fundamentals described in this book, like posture, and how your feet touch the ground, will be invaluable."

Bill Bilodeau
Recreational runner, barefoot and shod, 52 years old

"This thought provoking and easy to read book had me intrigued and tempted within minutes. It truly puts the burden of proof back on the running shoe industry!"

Chantelle Wilder
2009 Canada World Cross Country team
Runners Feed writer and co-owner
Former barefoot running skeptic

"Like most runners I know in their 40s, I am desperate to again be able to run healthy. I fought the central thesis of this book, but by addressing some of my main concerns again and again, Ashish has convinced me to try barefoot running."

Alex Tilson
American 50K record holder (2002-2009)

"I don't want to wear shoes. Why is there a book called Run Barefoot except if it is good for you?"

Greta Gunter
6 years wise

RUN **BAREFOOT** RUN **HEALTHY**

Less Pain More Gain For Runners Over 30

ASHISH MUKHARJI

Heterodox Press

ISBN 978-0-9830354-0-4

Library of Congress Control Number: 2011908794

Heterodox Press: info@heterodoxpress.com

Cover design by Vrbanac Zoltán.
Author photo by CreativeShot/Christophe Testi.
Illustrations by Symphonix Multimedia and Print/Paul Cox.
Book design by Symphonix Multimedia and Print/Justin Oefelein.

Photographs:

Page 43:   Splayed bare feet: Hoffman, Phil. 1905, Conclusions Drawn from a Comparative Study of Barefoot and Shoe-Wearing Peoples, The Journal of Bone and Joint Surgery, 1905;s2-3:p107.
Page 44:   Feet squashed by shoes, and the shoes: Ibid, p110.
Page 46:   Child grasping straw with foot: Ibid, p120.
Page 143:   Bare feet: Ibid, p108.
Page 144:   Aftermath of foot binding: Ibid, p113.
Page 48:   Photograph of Pons Fabricius by Matthias Kabel, licensed under the Creative Commons Attribution-Share Alike 3.0 Unported license.
Page 124:   Snapshot of treadmill video: courtesy Dr. Marc Silberman.

Table of Contents

And forget not that the earth delights to feel your bare feet and the winds long to play with your hair.

Khalil Gibran

Foreword

I have always run barefoot. My earliest memories of running are playing games with my cousins and I could always outrun them. Growing up in South Africa, it is just natural to go barefoot. My kids went to school barefoot and children are encouraged to do sport barefoot at junior level. It is an accepted medical fact that your foot muscles develop better if you do not wear any shoes. Growing up in Bloemfontein, South Africa, I was privileged to start training and running in a milieu of barefoot running. Most of my peers ran barefoot and the senior South African women's 100m and 200m record holder was also a barefoot runner. The first woman to break 2 minutes for 800m in South Africa ran barefoot as well as the first man to run under 4 minutes for the mile. Therefore it was not strange to run barefoot.

I just love the feel and freedom of running barefoot. It just feels different from running with heavy training shoes. I can recommend barefoot running as a way to get in touch with your body's intelligence because you are so aware of your running form and what is happening with and in your body.

Enjoy running as part of your life and let it enrich your daily existence. Get in touch with nature by going barefoot, and listen to your body while you are running. It will change your outlook on life profoundly.

Read this book.

ZOLA

Zola Budd Pieterse
Olympian
World Cross Country Champion (1985, 1986)
World Record Holder, 5000 meters (1985)

Acknowledgments

This was much more of a team project than I had originally envisioned.

For sharing their own barefoot stories, I am grateful to: Angela Bishop, Burt Malcuit, Tim Cunningham, Tamara Gerken, Cassie Howard, Owen McCall, Efrem Rensi, Julian Romero, John Stieber, and Heather Wiatrowski.

My thanks to the scientists and physicians who generously provided guidance and suggestions: Dr. Amy Adams, Prof. Dan Ariely, Dr. Ray McClanahan, Dr. Joseph Froncioni, Dr. Sherri Greene, Dr. Daniel Lieberman, Dr. Michael Nirenberg, Dr. Steven Robbins, Michael Warburton, and Dr. Bernhard Zipfel.

For their encouragement throughout the creative process, I am indebted to Reggie Solomon and Laura Joukovski. Without their generous help and deadlines, I'd still be writing.

For their assistance in shaping the text, I thank my readers: Shanda Bahles, Bill Bilodeau, Naomi Brown, Joel Davidson, Corinne DeBra, Vanessa Flynn, Mary Ann Furda, Jerry Harris, Kate Honan, Jon Kroll, Anu Mukharji-Gorski, Cynthia Neuwalder, Susan Ryan, Michelle Steed, and Ksenia Siegel, and my editor, Peter Gerardo.

Thanks to Charles Tripp for his technology help, and to David Every for technology assistance as well as his insights into the martial arts. Thanks also to Darcy Bliss, Tim Brennan, Dr. Mirella Bucci, Jim Haselmaier, Mark Sisson (marksdailyapple.com), and Darren Richardson, for their help connecting me to sources and research.

Thanks to Toddy Fitch, Clementine Gunter and Stefani van Wijk for their cover design inspiration, and to The Book Doctors, Arielle Eckstut and David Henry Sterry, for their guidance on delivering this book into your hands.

Thanks to my running buddies, occasional and regular: Christin Dilley, Amy Eastwood, Alex Gagnon, John Hatfield, Vinod Herur, Diego May, Vibeka Sen Sisodiya, Justin Sleasman, Laura Sleasman, the Dolphin South End Run Club, and the Palo Alto Run Club.

Last but not least, I am very grateful to all those who shared their barefoot running questions and experiences: Marie Altman, Shaily Bhargav, Jack Bascom, Bill Bilodeau, Vanessa Braunstein, Justin Boggs, Chris Calandro, Tracy Carver, Courtney Chalupa, Baylor Chapman, Hae Min Cho, Peter Coughlan, Joel Davidson, Corinne DeBra, Joe Dito, Ilsa Dohmen, Amy Eastwood, Elaine Eng, Taia Ergueta, Aleksander Fedorynski, Cornelia Fletcher, Emily Finch, Vanessa Flynn, Darshana Maya Greenfield, Sam Hariri, Don Hatch, Sam Holdsworth, Shanthi Iyer, Carol Kahl, Joe Kaniewski, Brad Kilpatrick, Koko, Roni Kornitz, Val Lisiewicz, Abby Lorenz, Roger Magoulas, Jeff Mazer, Mike McGehee, Peter McKenna, Jessica Merrill, Blake Mills, David Mineau, Amer Moorhead, David P. Moulton, Karen Mudurian, Dhiraj Mukherjee, Mohit Mukherjee, Kathy Overstreet, Rich Pasco, Richard Pearson, Jason Perez, Michelle Pualuan, Wendy Spies, Anya Starovoytov, Piyush Sevalia, Nicolas Sizaret, Don Strachan, Georgi Stoev, Valerie Stack, Laura Stec, Vidya Sundaram, Erwin Tenhumberg, Clarkia Thijsse, Anne Thomas, Chris Tilghman, Mani Varadarajan, Kristina Velarde, Wes Walker, Mike Wall, Jim Warhol, Scott Wharton, Bracken White, Kevin Wrynn, Kendall Wu, and Adam Ziemba.

Introduction

I've been running for almost a quarter-century. I still remember lacing up my very first pair of Nike Air Pegasus and heading up the fire trail to explore the hills above the Berkeley campus. Far from the hustle and bustle of college life, the view of San Francisco Bay and the Golden Gate Bridge was stunning, as it still is on a clear day.

Since that first tentative outing, running has provided me with many more spectacular vistas, as well as friends and adventures, runner's highs and good health, and shin splints, my constant companion.

To run is to please the doctors, who prescribe regular exercise along with veggies and Lipitor, as well as the statisticians, whose actuarial tables promise a few extra hours of life as reward for each sweaty workout.

But why must it hurt so much? "No pain, no gain," we're told. If it hurts, it must be working. Suck it up!

That's just what I did – through three marathons and several year-long, injury-induced layoffs.

Fast-forward 20 years. In early 2007, the ultra-running magazine *Marathon & Beyond* published an article on the advantages of running barefoot – without shoes. I must have been particularly frustrated by injury, because I sent back an angry postcard to the editor, asserting that only the genius of shoe researchers allowed me to keep running, however infrequently and painfully. How dare they question my lifeline to health!

Well, certainty is often a harbinger of change ahead. It took one more year, until the day running-induced pain reduced me to crawling around my apartment, that I realized I had turned the running-technology dial as far as it could go.

I haven't run in shoes since that day. Nor have I suffered my previously chronic shin splints, plantar fasciitis, or IT Band Syndrome. At age 41, sans shoes, I've returned to peak physical condition – to the good health that should have been mine all along, until technological "innovation" got in the way.

The experience of joyful, painless running is available to you too. I hope you enjoy reading about the natural miracle of barefoot running and that you'll join me on this path.

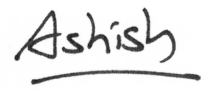

Note: Throughout the text, I cite scientific papers and helpful books, articles and videos. The tags PAPER1, VIDEO2, ARTICLE3, etc., lead to a bibliography in the back of the book.

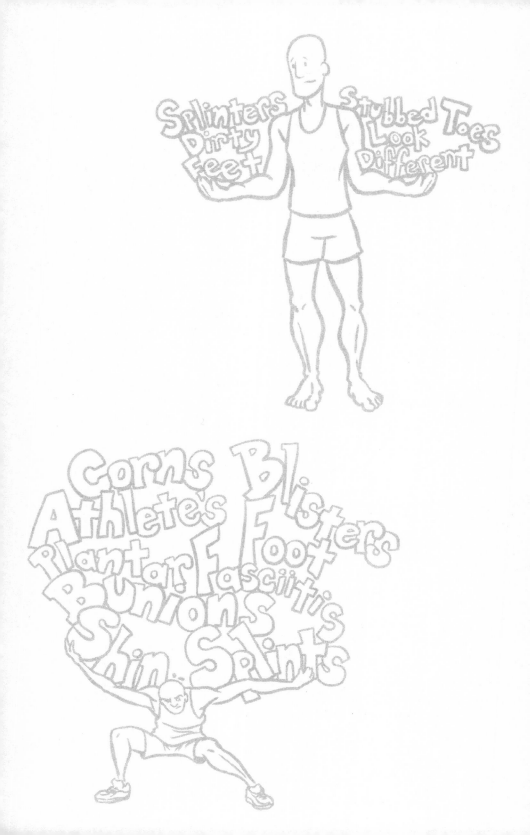

Is This For Real?

Is this for real?

Absolutely. [PAPER1] You can run barefoot. And you'll probably have a lot more fun.

Why on earth run barefoot?

Runners lose the shoes for three main reasons:
- To reduce chronic running injuries, including runner's knee, shin splints, plantar fasciitis and IT Band Syndrome.
- To rediscover the joy of running.
- To reduce cost.

Why would barefoot running be healthier? That sure seems counterintuitive.

Cushioned running shoes attempt to muffle the impact of running. In contrast, barefoot running reduces impact before it happens, by encouraging good running form.

Here's how it works. Our bodies depend on sensory input to move. Shoes reduce that sensory input. Like blindfolds on the feet, shoes reduce the body's proprioception (awareness of orientation in space) and fluidity of movement. Going barefoot restores sensory input and thereby improves our quality of movement.

In addition:
- Feet perform their natural function best when their shape and movement are uninhibited.
- Wearing shoes introduces a host of foot ailments that bare feet just don't get.

You don't actually mean "barefoot," do you? Or are you recommending those funky toe shoes? Surely my skin shouldn't touch the dirty ground!

I do mean skin to the ground. Run for exercise, run for your health, run for pleasure, on the roads, or wherever you prefer – barefoot as the day you were born.

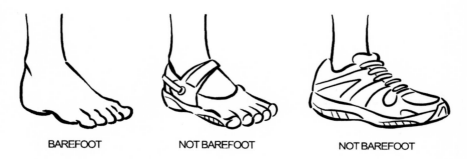

BAREFOOT   NOT BAREFOOT   NOT BAREFOOT

Think about this: why do we wear running shoes? We weren't born wearing shoes. For what purpose did we adopt them? What medical or scientific research led us to the hefty shoes we wear today?

What you'll discover is that no science exists to justify the design of the modern built-up running shoe, which constrains and changes the natural movement of your foot. I was incredulous, then shocked, and ultimately inspired as I grew to appreciate the functional beauty of the human foot. Perhaps your transition will be similar.

This would be a good time to point out that certain large corporations have co-opted the word "barefoot" to mean "running in our overpriced brand-name shoes." That is not what barefoot means.

Later, I'll go into more detail about shoes, but for now, please know that whenever I say "barefoot," I mean completely shoeless, as opposed to "shod" – wearing shoes.

Internet discussion boards are packed with stories of stress fractures in runners who wear "barefoot shoes." When I walk into a running store and overhear the chirpy salesperson tell an injured runner, "Let me show you our new barefoot running shoes," I want to scream.

Is running barefoot safe?

The human body evolved to run barefoot, and to this day, recreational runners complete marathon races (26.2 miles) barefoot. Yes, it's safe. More to the point, running barefoot is probably safer than running in bulky shoes.

Although most barefoot runners reduce their injury count, throwing away your running shoes does not grant you a cloak of invincibility. Before you rush out to run barefoot, read the chapters on running form and transitioning.

Is barefoot running painful?

Running on clean smooth pavement is great fun, once you get over the initial nervousness. For many of us, it opens up a new world of receiving sensations through the feet. Stepping on gravel and acorns does hurt, but the pain dissipates immediately. It won't keep you from running the next step, the next day, or well into old age.

Of course, stepping on broken beer bottles and other sharp objects is unpleasant. Fortunately, puncture wounds are rare, and heal quickly. (More about this in the Injury chapter.)

What about cushioning? I know I need cushioning.

A few years ago, I had some work done on my guitar by a repairman working from his garage. I noticed that the walls of his workspace were adorned with posters for Mixed Martial Arts (MMA). I remarked, backing away slowly, "This is some violent stuff you have here!" He replied that

MMA wasn't violent at all: fighters are bare-knuckled or wear very light gloves, and bouts last only a few minutes till skin breaks and blood is drawn.

By contrast, he continued, contestants in the "gentlemanly" sport of boxing wear padded gloves to reduce superficial skin injuries, allowing their brains to get bounced around their skulls for as many as 12 rounds.

Would you rather have a bruised pinkie or a concussed brain?

The situation with running shoes is much the same. Yes, shoes eliminate the occasional "owie" from stepping on acorns. But by numbing the natural feedback from your feet, padded shoes provide a false sense of security, and permit – even encourage – unnatural pounding that penetrates your legs and back, leading to chronic injuries and long-term damage.

You mention injuries. Is jogging bad for you?

Jogging implies a jerky, jarring, up-and-down motion. That's not ideal. Henceforth, we are all "runners."

Running, whatever the pace, should involve a smooth, flowing motion. You want to feel quick and light on your feet.

That's best achieved when your feet can feel the ground, and they self-adapt to make the lightest possible contact with the ground.

What do I need to know before running barefoot?

When we were children, running barefoot came naturally. It doesn't require any specialized knowledge. I provide guidance on form and transitioning, but all you really need to know is this: just go out there, be relaxed, and enjoy it!

Let's say for the sake of argument that the human body evolved to run barefoot. But that was in nature, right? Surely we weren't designed to run on hard concrete and asphalt. Isn't running barefoot on roads worse than wearing comfy cushioned shoes?

Any experienced barefoot runner will tell you that a clean, smooth, asphalt road is the Cadillac of surfaces. Read the interview with barefoot runner Efrem Rensi.

"Natural" surfaces do not look like the 18th Hole at Pebble Beach. Natural surfaces are uneven, can be just as hard as asphalt, and may contain divots and hidden sharp objects.

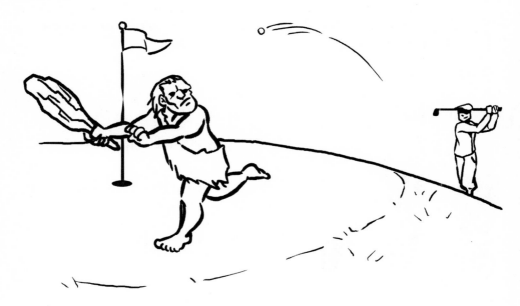

Our distant ancestors could run almost anywhere. Today, our Western feet have been tenderized by years of wearing shoes, so most of us will find it easier to start out running barefoot on clean roads than through the African savanna.

What was the life expectancy of those distant ancestors? 25? 30? Why should I follow their example?

Don't run barefoot "because" your ancestors were barefoot. Consider losing the shoes because:

▸ Despite (or because of?) years of wearing modern footwear, your feet and legs still suffer chronic aches or more serious injuries, and

▸ As you keep reading, you realize that society's move to shoes, and the design of modern built up running shoes, was driven by culture and fashion, not function.

What are the health benefits of barefoot running?

For me, the main benefit of barefoot running has been a sharp reduction in chronic injuries: shin splints, plantar fasciitis and IT Band Syndrome. And that's while running farther and faster than I did while shod.

Many runners, who may have switched to barefoot running to reduce injuries, also enjoy the feeling of being in a more natural state – connected directly to the earth.

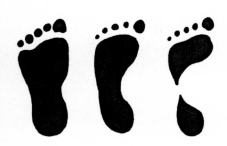

Runners with "high arches" or "flat feet" often report that their feet regain normal, healthy, strong arches.

And it's just plain more fun.

Even if being barefoot is healthier for those who've always done it, can Westerners who've lived in shoes safely make the transition?

Absolutely. Thousands are doing it. It's like giving up smoking. You can always adopt a healthier lifestyle, though it may take a few months.

Listen to your body, follow my guidelines in the transition chapter, and take it as slowly and gently as you need.

Must runners sacrifice comfort for long-term benefit?

Most barefoot runners enjoy and prefer running barefoot – it's not a penance. The word "joy" keeps popping up in my interviews.

Your feet, too, may prefer being bare to being crammed into chafing, stinky, sweat-soaked running shoes. Try it.

How far can I run barefoot?

You can run as long and as far as your feet feel comfortable. Once your feet have adapted, there's no inherent limit.

In marathon training, I run over 50 miles per week barefoot, without any foot issues. I am much more likely to feel tired from a hard workout, or feel the burn of chafing skin elsewhere on my body, than to have any pain in my feet. They are so much happier being free to breathe and to move.

If this is so great, why aren't more people doing it?

More people are doing it every day. And I hope that with better education about the consequences of built-up running shoes, many more will experience the health benefits and pleasures of barefoot running.

This all sounds interesting, but I don't see myself running barefoot. Maybe minimalist. Should I keep reading, or donate this book to the library?

Keep reading. You can still benefit from the guidance on running form and injury prevention, as well as the interviews with runners and podiatrists.

Is barefoot running appropriate for all ages, including children?

Yes. Children have excellent running form until they pick up bad habits from their adults. Many of my friends reminisce about running on gravel when they were young – an ability most of us have lost.

In his wonderful book *Impro,* acting teacher Keith Johnstone writes that rather than think of children as immature adults, he began to see adults as atrophied children.

If you have children, you know how they can comfortably hold all those twisty yoga poses that defy our best grown-up efforts. Children use their bodies naturally and efficiently, until adults get in the way. Don't get in the way.

Won't their delicate feet get hurt by sharp objects?

NYC podiatrist Sherri Greene says that while we need to be aware of broken glass and other dangers of the urban environment, "I think it is great to keep children barefoot to allow the bones to grow, the muscles to get stronger and the ligaments to strengthen naturally. I think children being barefoot is super positive for them. You don't want to restrict the foot at all."

You might also read the classic book, *Take off Your Shoes and Walk*, by podiatrist Simon Wikler. [BOOK1]

Don't we need more support in our shoes?

Doing away with cushioned heel-raised running shoes reduces the risk of injury. Hard to believe at first, but as you'll read, it is true.

The human foot has evolved over millions of years to support our moving bodies with ease and fluidity. Rigid, restrictive shoes with raised heels interfere with that natural movement. Modern shoes attempt to change or even replace the function of the foot. Unsurprisingly, they fail.

Your best bet is to let the body do what it does best, without getting in the way. Please be sure to read the interviews with podiatrists Dr. Ray McClanahan and Dr. Michael Nirenberg, as well as Dr. Philip Hoffman's paper. [PAPER14]

Our entire generation has been led by advertising to believe that we need more "support" in our shoes. This claim is not supported by any scientific evidence.

When and where did this fad of barefoot running begin?

Pet rocks were a fad. Rubik's Cube was a fad. Wearing baggy pants below the butt is a fad.

Humans ran barefoot for millennia before the invention of shoes, and in particular, before the invention in the 1970s of bulky modern running shoes. Barefoot running has always been with us, and it's here to stay.

Why are you rejecting all the advances of modern technology?

I'm a big fan of useful technology, such as my GPS watch, moisture-wicking running fabrics, and chip timing on race day. I certainly see why supportive running shoes might have seemed a good technology to try – much like hydrogenated fats as an alternative to butter. But like those hydrogenated fats, it's time to deep six the idea that built-up running shoes are either necessary or desirable.

Considerable anecdotal evidence, and a large and growing body of scientific literature (detailed in the following chapters), tell us that supportive shoes are bad, bad, bad.

Easy for you to say. You probably have a super symmetrical and athletic body.

No. My family tree does not list any athletic accomplishments, and I've never been on a sports team, even in grade school. No matter what your athletic status, I've probably been more injured (and more often) than you have.

I run barefoot because it's much easier on my aging, creaky body. If you suffer running injuries, going barefoot will likely be easier on your body, too.

Will people think I'm poor if I run barefoot?

People used to associate bare feet with poverty and "living on the wrong side of the tracks." But given all the attention that barefoot running is getting these days, they might just think that you're brilliant.

Why have you written this book?

I'm American. Inactivity, obesity, and the resulting poor health are epidemic in this country, and unnecessarily so.

The good health we derive from running – that most basic and inexpensive form of exercise – is available to everyone. I get so frustrated when I hear, "I can't run because my knees hurt," or "I gave up running when my back began to hurt," because I know that in so many cases, *the root of the problem isn't with the knees or back, but with the footwear.*

For my reader, particularly the injured reader who might think that running is forever out of reach, I hope that barefoot running will open up the possibility of regular exercise and a longer and healthier life.

Write to me at ashish@runbarefootrunhealthy.com with your success stories!

Summary: Barefoot running is a normal, natural activity, providing more enjoyment and greater health for all.

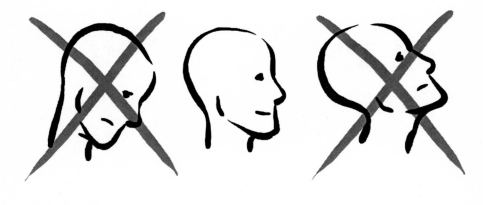

Remember: Keep A Neutral Neck

Meet The Author

And you are ...?

I'm a middle-of-the-pack runner, learning how to run injury-free and stay healthy.

So this barefoot thing works for you. Well, aren't you special?

It seems to work for most runners who make the switch. In fact, it works for all the barefoot runners I know. And these are runners who had accumulated many injuries while running in shoes.

What qualifies you to write on this topic?

I have been running for over 20 years, and have run five marathons, including two barefoot marathons. In addition to my personal experience transitioning from "injured yet again" to running 70 barefoot miles per week, I corresponded with many of the world's leading foot and running researchers (see the Science chapter for links to their work), and researched over 100 years of scientific literature to assemble this book.

However, I haven't always believed in barefoot running. As I wrote in the introduction, although chronically injured through much of my running career, I felt indebted to my beefy running shoes. Fortunately, *Marathon & Beyond* did not publish my angry response to their article on barefoot running, or I'd be writing under a pen name today.

Only after many years sidelined by injury did I make the connection that as my running shoes got bigger and more expensive, my injuries just got worse.

From my experience, I learned to question my assumptions, and I trust that others can do the same.

So you found a method that works for you. Great. Why try to convert others?

I hate to see my friends, some as young as teenagers, injured and couch-bound when they should be thriving.

I'm frustrated at the growing campaign of fear and misinformation – for instance, open letters from CEOs of major shoe manufacturers and retailers – warning of dire consequences should runners try to go barefoot. Call me an idealist.

Okay, let's step back a minute. You said you used to like your shoes. How did you get into barefoot running?

Over a 20-year, non-competitive running career, I was injured about two-thirds of the time: plantar fasciitis, Achilles tendonitis, chronic shin splints, runner's knee, IT Band Syndrome, back and neck pain … I've had it all.

I tried a variety of orthotics, expensive physical therapy, Rolfing, exquisitely painful deep-tissue massage, ever-heavier and more expensive running shoes, and I could barely keep my running injuries in check well enough to run four times a week.

With each year, the injuries got worse. I couldn't run more than two days in a row. An ill-conceived track workout at the local high school left me in such pain that I was crawling to get around the house.

That led to crutches and the hospital. I recently requested my medical records from that hospital visit. My podiatrist was a former president of the California Board of Podiatric Medicine. His written words are just as I remember them: I should "... slowly get back to running heel-to-toe style. Recommended Superfeet type device ..."

In other words, more of the same. There had to be another way.

I notice you live in California. Are you some kind of hippie?

My degree is in mathematics. I believe in following the data. In the case of barefoot running, theory, data and personal experience seem to align very well.

I provide a summary and links to the best available science on the topic. You can read the abstracts and request the papers yourself. Running barefoot requires no belief other than a willingness to try something new, and to trust the feedback from your own two feet.

Here's what my shoe-wearing non-hippie friend Dave recently emailed me after our lunchtime discussion of barefoot running:

> "For what it's worth, I have to admit our discussion changed my views a lot. I started by thinking not that you're silly or anything - just kinda the earthy/back-to-nature stuff that some of my friends have. (Not that there's anything wrong with that). But after talking with you, and knowing enough about physical therapy and over-training, etc., I came away thinking it probably is a much safer way to train (for non competitive running)."

How far do you run barefoot?

I don't have a fixed plan. Most weeks, I run between 20 and 70 miles, with long runs of up to 22 miles.

The key is this: I run when I feel like it. My running is dictated by my mood and schedule, and is no longer limited by my injuries. You have the same potential.

How many days per week do you run?

I typically run five or six days a week. The missed days are when life gets in the way – not injuries. I can't tell you what a change that is from my shod days. Again, when I ran in shoes, my shin splints usually prevented me from running more than two days in a row, or more than four times a week.

You never ran three days in a row with shoes?

As I sat in the dentist's chair a few years ago, my hygienist, Amy, mentioned that she ran every morning before work. "Every morning!" I thought. "That's great! I've gotta do that!" So I did – for one week. I was then laid up for a month with the worst shin splints of my life.

Why should I listen to you? You aren't an elite runner.

True. This is not a book of, by or for elite runners. I weigh a lot more than 130 pounds, I don't have a shoe company sponsorship, I don't have perfect biomechanics, and I don't have a team of trainers, massage therapists and doctors to tend to my every twinge. Do you?

This is a book for the rest of us, who must juggle our busy lives with a running program that will keep us fit enough to navigate life's adventures into old age.

And since you mention it, many of those shod elite runners have endured significant injuries and multiple surgeries.

You want me to disregard everything I know, and put my trust in you?

No. No one person has all the answers, and I don't either. Whenever I read a book or article on a topic I know well, I'm amazed how many details are incorrect. So, don't put all your faith in a single source, even this one.

I *do* hope that you'll consider the advice and facts presented here, follow some of the links to published, peer-reviewed research, and trust the feedback from your own body to guide your decision.

Trust *yourself.* Don't give in to fear and advertising.

How has running helped your health?

The other day I had a "mini-physical" before my regular blood donation. After three straight weeks with long runs of about 20 miles, I had my best blood pressure and pulse readings ever. Exercise can get sweaty, but it really works.

Will I need surgery if I run barefoot?

My personal goal is to keep running 'til the day I die of old age, avoiding surgery along the way. Barefoot running provides no guarantee against surgeries and illness, but it does help maintain a healthy lifestyle. It's good for the body and easy on the legs.

Barefoot running can't eliminate all knee issues, but by reducing the forces on your knees, it can reduce the risk. [PAPER12]

Do you run races? Is this just for competitive runners?

I run mainly to stay healthy. A race or two a year is a nice motivator and fitness check.

My personal running goal is to qualify for the Boston Marathon. I was trying to run faster in order to qualify, but now I think I should just get older, since the qualifying bar drops every five years!

You need not be a racer to benefit from barefoot running. You need only have the goal of good health. I can't stress it enough: "winning" is about staying healthy, not about standing on some podium.

Did you grow up barefoot? What about the rest of us who grew up wearing shoes?

I grew up wearing typical sneakers with raised heels.

Summary: I'm no elite athlete. I feel your pain. That's why I recommend running barefoot.

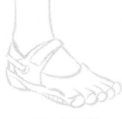

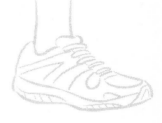

BAREFOOT   NOT BAREFOOT   NOT BAREFOOT

Meet The Podiatrist:
Dr. Ray McClanahan

And you are ...?

Dr. McClanahan: Dr. Ray McClanahan. I am a podiatrist and podiatric surgeon practicing at the Northwest Foot & Ankle Clinic in Portland, Oregon. I am also an active runner and athlete; my PR [personal record] in the 5,000 meters is 13:56, and I qualified for the World Duathlon Championships in 2001.

Dr. McClanahan, you have a lot of experience with feet and running. Why run barefoot?

Dr. McClanahan: Based on my experience of seeing running injuries and based on evaluations of barefoot cultures, I think running barefoot enables some individuals to decrease the number of musculoskeletal injuries that they would experience were they to run in conventional running shoes.

I also have not found in my 15 years of podiatry practice that any manmade technology can overcome or supersede the natural ability of the human foot in locomotion.

So my own personal experience suggests running barefoot is a path to better, more natural biomechanics.

Is there research on the topic of barefoot versus shod running?

Dr. McClanahan: There's actually quite a bit done by Dr. Daniel Lieberman at Harvard. Not only has he published in the journal *Nature*, he's also got some sophisticated video analysis [VIDEO4] showing the differences between what happens when you slam down on the ground with a huge heel versus what happens when you lightly touch down on the ground with a bare foot.

I spent some of my growing up years in Africa. As an adolescent, I witnessed firsthand that people can perform at very high levels of athleticism without shoes.

So, I think just being able to see people functioning well without shoes is enough compelling evidence for me. I don't need a research project to tell me what I can physically see.

Surely, one thing that shoes give us is arch support. How can we do without arch support?

Dr. McClanahan: I've had lots of conversations with physicists and architects and engineers and people who've built bridges, and they tell me that when they build bridges, what enables the bridge to carry the load is having both support ends flat and level.

I tell my patients, "Yes, you want arch support, but you want your *own* arch to support your body, and that is accomplished by having your heel completely level with the ball of the foot out to the end of the toes."

Yet when you look at most running shoes, this rule is violated at both support ends: the back support end is always at least an inch higher than the front, and the more recent toe-spring feature takes the front part of the arch and artificially elevates it above the support surface.

I hold my foot in that heel-raised position in the clinic, and I show patients what happens when I bear weight on such a configuration: the open space begins to collapse. In other words, the foot goes into pronation, and the arch begins to fall.

I tell runners that if they want arch support, it doesn't require putting something under the arch. That violates physical principles. That's not how an arch functions.

The only way an arch functions is for the heel to be completely level with all the toes. In other words, it's the same position that you would see on your own bare foot when you bear weight: your heel is level with the front of your foot.

Do you think that being barefoot is safe for children and their developing feet?

Dr. McClanahan: I do. In fact, it would be better if we started in our childhood. I try to get parents to encourage their children to go barefoot, and when they're not barefoot, to encourage them to be in a shoe that would let them have their foot positioned as if it were barefoot.

You got the letter from a running retailer warning of nails and beer bottles and pea-sized pebbles lying in ambush. What about the risk of serious injury?

Dr. McClanahan: As a barefoot runner myself, and having watched barefoot runners transition, I would say the fear is significantly overblown. I don't think puncturing your foot happens as often to barefoot runners as the majority of the population would assume.

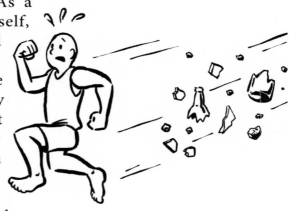

Shoes create their own problems. The Badwater Ul-tramarathon is a 135-mile race across Death Valley. I saw a video interview of the previous champion. They showed him putting his shoes on, and he had no toenails. So the interviewer said, "I notice you don't have any toenails. What happened there?" And his response was, "I had my toenails removed so I could wear running shoes."

He said it without batting an eye. He said it as if that's what you have to do if you're going to wear running shoes.

One of my friends and I were watching the video, and we rolled around with laughter because people don't even see the absurdity of what we're doing to ourselves with shoes.

Where can interested readers learn more about foot health?

Dr. McClanahan: I've written a number of articles on foot health and footwear choice, available on my website: www.nwFootAnkle.com.

Summary: Barefoot running enables better biomechanics.

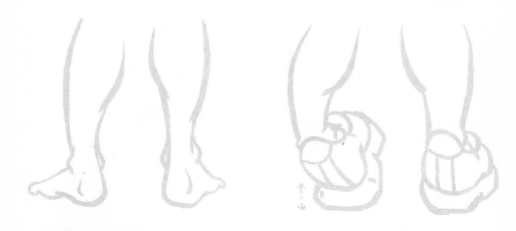

Who Can Run Barefoot?

Who can run barefoot?

Anyone who can run, can run barefoot. Even many people who think they can't run, can run barefoot if they try.

Christopher McDougall's *Born to Run* is a must-read for any athlete. He lays out a persuasive case that humans evolved to run long distances. It's what we were designed to do, to survive, long before modern running shoes and their advertising.

This isn't just true for skinny Africans. Human biomechanics are much more similar than different, no matter where you were born. And the modern published research on barefoot running has primarily been in the West.

I'm overweight. Is barefoot running appropriate for me?

Check with your physician. If your health does not preclude running altogether, then you can run barefoot.

The more you weigh, the greater the impact of running incorrectly, and the greater the benefit of adopting a flowing, barefoot-running style.

I have hip and knee issues. Is barefoot running appropriate for me?

Running barefoot is a lower (yes, lower!) impact sport than shod running, so it often reduces or eliminates chronic injuries and pain. Read my interviews with other barefoot runners.

Many runners have irreparable damage to the natural shock absorbers in their knees. Can running barefoot help them, or is it too late?

If you can run, you can probably run better barefoot. Running barefoot should reduce the impact and rotational forces on your knees. [PAPER2] [PAPER12] Give it a try, take it easy, and listen to your body.

If your knees are already damaged from years of pounding in shoes, don't continue with more of the same!

I can't address the specifics of your knees, but science tells us that glucosamine/chondroitin can provide some help to worn out knees. [PAPER16]

I overpronate. Can I run barefoot?

Before "overpronation" became a medical diagnosis requiring expensive shoes and medical care, "pronation" was a natural movement pattern, useful for preventing injury. [PAPER6]

As you'll read, shoes with raised heels and stiff soles first hurt us by causing excessive pronation and then hurt us by artificially blocking the movement of the foot.

I have high arches. Can I run barefoot?

Many runners with high arches find that their feet take a healthier form, with picture-perfect arches, after just a few months of running barefoot. With use, previously atrophied muscles regain much of their natural strength.

Start out slowly, follow the guidelines laid out here, and *always* listen to your body.

I have Morton's neuroma. Can I run barefoot?

Yes you can. Read the interview with Barefoot TJ.

When I run more than a mile, I feel a very sharp pain on the side of my knees. I've been told it is Iliotibial Band Syndrome (ITBS). I couldn't possibly do without the cushioning.

Here's the deal: you don't need more cushioning. You need to put less strain on your legs in the first place. The best way to do that is to stop heel striking. *Be a wheel, not a pogo-stick.*

ITBS plagued me for more than 10 years, and it completely sidelined me for three. One time, 15 miles into a NYC Marathon training run, ITBS kicked in, stranding me five miles from home. I couldn't run more than a step without agonizing pain. My guardian angel must have been looking out for me that day, as a friend just happened to drive past, see me sadly limping home, and give me a ride.

Nowadays, I run much farther, and since I started running barefoot, ITBS has never recurred.

The sole of my foot hurts terribly. My doctor says I have plantar fasciitis (PF). He wants to inject me with steroids, and surgery may be in my future. I couldn't possibly do without the cushioning.

I had PF. I had a steroid injection, and I was threatened with surgery. No more. Many other barefoot runners tell similar stories of "miraculous" recovery. Read the interviews.

Before steroids and surgery, don't you owe it to yourself to try every alternative?

I have one flat and one high-arched foot. Can I run barefoot?

Yes.

I have one prosthetic leg. Can I run barefoot?

I don't see why not. The length of the prosthetic leg (and shoe, if any) should more or less match the length of your bare foot, and some special concerns may apply. For instance, be careful not to bang the edge of your prosthesis against your good foot.

I have shin splints. I couldn't possibly do without the cushioning.

I had chronic shin splints for years, 24/7. They're gone.

In runners, shin splints seem to be caused by the raised heel and by cushioning that leads to a harder pounding. Running barefoot eliminates both causes. Try it!

I hurt my hip. Can I run barefoot?

As with all other injuries, first be kind to your body. Give yourself time to rest and recover. When you think you're ready to run, run barefoot. You may find that injuries caused by the impact of shod running no longer occur.

I just run for fun. I don't need to get so intense about this.

If you're satisfied with your running routine, and injuries aren't getting in the way, I wouldn't expect you to change a thing.

I'm 25 years old. Why is this reserved for "over 30 runners"? Can't I run barefoot?

In my opinion, you can and should run barefoot. However, most 25-year-olds are too young to know the pain of chronic injury, and may be more focused on achieving peak performance today than on thinking about long-term health. Since you're reading this book, give barefoot running a try. It should help your enjoyment of the sport, and your wallet, as well as your race-day performance.

I'm 43. I'm too old to start running barefoot.

Not at all.

If injury keeps you from running, then you're the perfect age to make a change for the better. Many others started running barefoot when they were older than you. Even if you're in your 50s or 60s, you can run barefoot, and you certainly won't be the oldest barefoot runner.

Please read the interview with 60-year old John Stieber.

My back hurts when I run. I couldn't possibly do without the cushioning.

Again, running barefoot reduces impact forces on your body. Assuming that you don't have an acute back injury that makes any exercise dangerous, you're the perfect candidate for barefoot running.

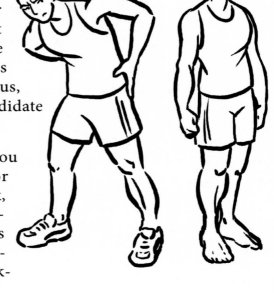

As an aside, if you suffer from pain or tightness in your back, or pretty much any-where from your hips to your neck, I encourage you to try Feldenk-rais. [RESOURCE2]

My legs are different lengths. Can I run barefoot?

Yes. I've also been told by doctors and physical thera-pists that my legs are different lengths, and I was prescribed orthotics. (I've also been told that my legs are *not* differ-ent lengths.) The orthotics didn't help, and neither did various shoe inserts. Losing the running shoes helped!

Unlike walking, the beauty of running is that you are not con-tacting the ground with both feet at the same time, so a length dis-crepancy, in the unlike-ly event you have one, shouldn't leave you running lopsided.

My neck hurts when I run. I couldn't possibly do without the cushioning.

Running barefoot reduces impact. In addition to the impact from pounding pavement, you may be holding tension in your neck. Try Alexander Technique. [RESOURCE1]

Should I run barefoot if I am currently suffering from a foot issue such as foot fungus or ingrown/missing toenails?

Foot fungus and missing toenails shouldn't keep you from running barefoot. If anything, allowing your feet to air out as you run barefoot may be beneficial.

Under what circumstances should I not do this?

If a doctor has advised you that running is dangerous to your health, take that advice or seek a second opinion from another physician. Also, if you're middle aged or older, you might want to consult a physician before beginning any new exercise program.

When you see the doctor, feel free to take along the list of scientific studies in the back of the book.

I always wear shoes, even at home. Can I run barefoot?

If your feet are completely unaccustomed to being bare, you may want to walk around the house barefoot for a few months, allowing your feet to regain some of their natural form and strength, before beginning the transition program.

Removing your outdoor shoes and going barefoot at home is more sanitary as well as healthier, whether or not you decide to run barefoot.

I work for a shoe company – can I run barefoot?

If you take the plunge, I commend you for your integrity and courage, and I also recommend the job-hunting website AskTheHeadhunter.com.

Summary: Barefoot running can benefit all runners.

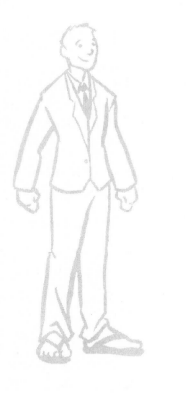
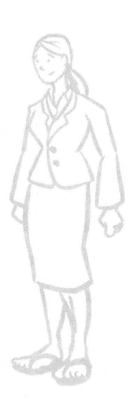

What About My Feet?

What about my feet? How are habitually bare feet different from habitually shod feet?

In 1905, Dr. Philip Hoffman wrote a very readable paper on foot health, available for free on the Web [PAPER14], and still considered a classic work. Hoffman worked at a time when many cultures still lived without shoes. He examined bare feet that had never worn shoes, witnessed their transition to shoes, and discussed the changes. I'll quote some of his observations, and I encourage you to read his original writings. His is the most eloquent description I've read of the damage caused by shoes.

In the picture below [PAPER14, p4], note the width of a natural forefoot, and the spread and direction of the toes.

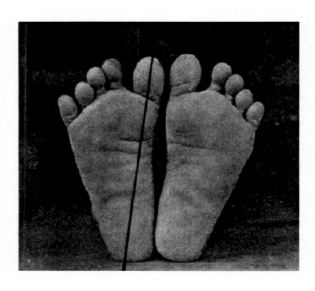

From that wide-toed start, look what happens to the human foot when you cram it into a pair of shoes [PAPER14, p7]:

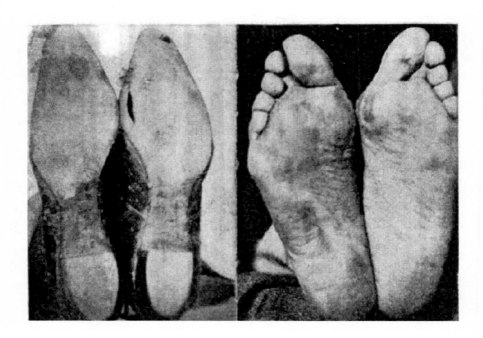

No matter what a shoe company executive might say about the dangers of going barefoot, is it not clear that something is very wrong in the pictures above?

How much thicker does the barefoot runner's skin get, compared to a city walker who never takes his shoes off?

Research published in 1931 noted that the coriums (soles) of Bantu natives in South Africa were between 6 and 9mm thick – as much as a third of an inch! [PAPER7]

During the years I've been running barefoot, the skin on the soles of my feet has thickened, and I suspect the bones have as well. The difference is not that perceptible, and the thickness of my soles is nowhere near a third of an inch.

To enjoy running and stay injury free, I don't focus on physical changes in my body. My attention is on the *use* of my body, on the sensations I feel through my feet, and on maintaining a tall-yet-relaxed posture and a fluid motion.

You tell me not to think about my soles, but I know they are very sensitive.

True. Throughout history, a favorite method of torture has been the bastinado or falanga – caning the soles of the feet to cause agonizing pain while leaving no mark.

But running barefoot is not comparable to someone caning your feet. When you run barefoot, you run *differently* than when you run in shoes, particularly padded shoes.

If you never wear shoes, do the feet get wider? If so, do the bones get bigger or the muscles flatter?

Running barefoot, even as an adult, encourages your feet to revert to their natural form. So yes, many barefoot runners do report wider feet.

After my last running injury (when I was still wearing running shoes), I had an x-ray taken of my feet. I've run barefoot since then, so I'll have to get another x-ray to see whether the bones are noticeably thicker today.

Will the skin on my feet become unattractive and rough to the touch?

The skin on my feet is slightly thicker than before, but it's neither hard nor rough.

In fact, the most common reaction I get from strangers who ask to see or touch my feet is, "It's not rough at all!"

What may happen, though, is that you'll regain some of the natural function of your feet. To quote Hoffman: "In most adult shoe-wearers the toes, beyond giving additional length to the foot, are practically functionless, while in bare-footed peoples they serve a variety of functions, as in climbing and grasping." [PAPER14, p.14]

He goes on to say, "My attention was especially attracted to the condition of the skin covering the primitive foot; to a remarkable degree it resembles that of the hand. The skin of the sole is thick and tough, though very pliable, and free from the callous spots due to the continued friction of the boot, common in shoe-wearers." [PAPER14, pp.120-121]

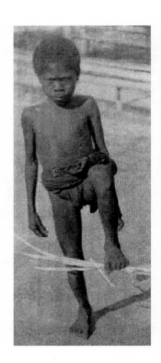

Will my feet become hard?

Think of the difference between muscles that are atrophied from disuse (an arm or leg in a cast) and muscles that are healthy from normal use. *That* transformation is what you can expect to see in your feet.

How will my sensitive soles adjust to going barefoot?

The sensitivity of your soles is actually an asset, not a liability. When you're just starting, your skin will let you know how long to run and when you need to stop. Stopping because of sensitive skin will prevent you from overburdening the foot muscles and tendons, initially atrophied from disuse. [PAPER13]

Any substances useful for toughening up the feet?

This isn't necessary. Your feet will become tougher over time, as they revive and gain strength from use.

Over the years, I've experimented with creams to soften or toughen my feet, but I don't think they did much. On the other hand, your feet do work hard for you, and massaging cream into them can feel like a treat. Do it for that reason, if you wish.

Bunions and corns. Gross!

Much of the grossness we associate with feet – smell, fungus, bunions and corns – is caused by cooping them up in tight, chafing, hot, damp, germ-infested foot-coffins. When you run in bare feet, the soles will get dirty (the dirt washes off), but your feet will look stronger and healthier. They will not stink or become misshapen. Your feet will look, smell and feel as they were meant to, and you'll be much more comfortable.

We hide our feet because we think they are gross. The truth is, they're only gross *because* we hide them! [PAPER11]

I have orthotics. Unless you have a suggestion to glue the orthotics to my bare feet, this is all irrelevant to me.

Over the years, well meaning doctors have prescribed me several different pairs of orthotics. Other doctors suggested hard inserts. I tried all of these. My feet and knees still hurt. When I got rid of the orthotics, the inserts and finally the shoes … only *then* did I get better.

Do you have enough arch support?

Your feet need arch support like a fish needs a bicycle.

Have you visited Europe? There, you'll find Roman bridges still standing after more than 2,000 years.

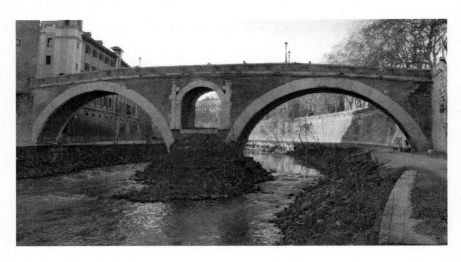

What supports the arches of those bridges? Nothing. Do you think the arch of a Roman bridge would be stronger if it were propped up by a jack – the way motion control running shoes, or expensive inserts, claim to support your feet? Of course not!

A well-designed arch gains strength as pressure is applied from above. Why would you explode the arch by applying force from below? (For more on this, please read the interview with Dr. McClanahan.)

My legs hurt until I got an arch insert.

The pain would also subside (temporarily) if you used crutches. But crutches aren't a long-term solution.

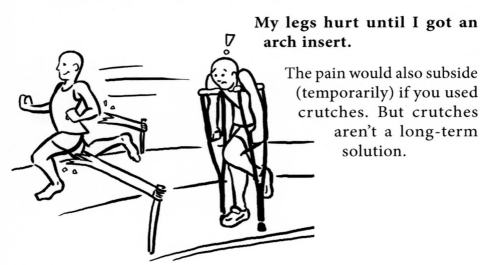

How do I take care of my feet when I get a cut or puncture?

Cuts on the sole of your foot are much less frequent than you'd think. In almost three years of running barefoot, I've suffered only a couple of minor cuts. I've never gotten a cut that kept me from finishing my run or from running the next day.

If you *do* get a cut, clean it with disinfectant and let it heal. Don't run on an open cut. If that means taking a couple of days off, take a couple of days off.

The nightly news would have us believe that disaster lurks around every corner, waiting to pounce if we're not safe in our SUVs, wearing bulky running shoes and perhaps a football helmet. This fear keeps us buying whatever TV advertisers are selling – even though most of us aren't in a war zone.

Rather than living in constant fear of the worst-case scenario, staying in tune with our bodies and surroundings will lead to better outcomes for most people, most of the time. And yes, wear your seatbelt.

You're saying no one has ever had a serious foot injury from running barefoot?

Serious foot injuries are extremely rare. Specifically, they are much more rare than the acute and chronic injuries that most shod runners experience as a matter of course. And which they don't think to blame on the real culprit: their shoes.

Do you run on an open sore?

I've never had a running-induced sore. If you have an open sore from some other condition, it's best to consult your physician and allow your body some healing rest.

I have flat feet with no spring to my arch. Wouldn't barefoot running be wrong for me?

Countless runners with formerly "flat feet" rediscovered their arches when they began running barefoot. This business of "flat feet" and "high arches" seems to be an artifact of modern shoes. Take away the shoes, and feet invariably regain their healthy form.

In his study of bare-footed peoples, Dr. Hoffman had a lot to say about the arch. For example: "The height and shape of the longitudinal arch have no bearing on the strength or usefulness of the foot. Weakness of the arch is rarely, if ever, accompanied by breaking or lowering, and *flat foot* as a *pathological* entity hardly exists." [Emphasis in the original.] [PAPER14, p. 32]

Read my eight interviews with real-life barefoot runners, who describe their prior injuries and their transition from shod to barefoot running.

Are you saying we shouldn't wear shoes altogether?

Some people do say that, but I don't see shoes disappearing from our society any time soon. When not running barefoot, try to wear shoes that allow your feet to maintain their natural form and movement. Avoid wearing heavy shoes with rigid soles and raised heels.

What exercises do you recommend to prepare my feet for running barefoot?

Once you are comfortable walking around your house barefoot, no further preparation is necessary. Find a clean, hard surface, and run only as long as it feels good. Barefoot running is not that complicated. In fact, it's very simple.

How do I prepare my otherwise bare feet for running shoes?

If you must occasionally run in shoes, no special preparation is necessary. Try to practice the good form you learned running barefoot. Good form is the key.

Over time, your feet may gradually widen to their natural size, so be sure to choose shoes that do not constrict them. You may need to shop for shoes with a wider forefoot than you have worn in the past.

What else can I do for my feet?

I enjoy rolling my feet on a golf ball as I sit at my desk. Trade foot massages with other barefoot runners - you'll figure out what feels good. (Remember, when you run barefoot, your feet may look a little dirty, but they won't sweat or stink.)

When not running, what kind of footwear is best?

Whenever possible, wear shoes without rigid soles and without raised heels. From a foot health point of view, it might be best if moccasins were to come back into style.

Will barefoot running give my feet calluses?

If you run with good form, the soles of your feet will get thicker – like soft leather. They shouldn't develop hard calluses.

I occasionally get hard calluses and hot spots after running a race. That's a sure sign that I pushed myself too hard and my running form deteriorated. Poor form will lead to injury, which is one reason I strongly advise new barefoot runners to avoid racing for at least one full season.

Summary: Your feet much prefer to be barefoot.

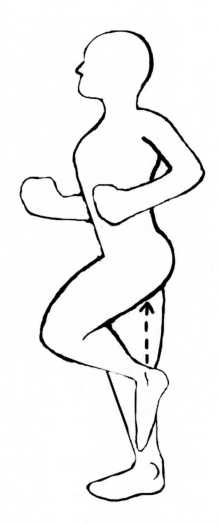

Remember: Lift Your Feet

But I Like Shopping For Shoes!

But I like shopping for shoes!

I know what you mean. From my pre-barefoot running days, I own seven pairs of Puma H Street shoes, all in bright colors that I can mix and match. I miss retail therapy, and I miss wearing my collection of colorful shoes and socks.

But I don't miss the shin splints, the plantar fasciitis and the IT Band Syndrome.

Could you possibly direct the impulse elsewhere – or at least toward shoes that don't have rigid soles and built-up heels? Running shoes with raised heels and rigid arch supports throw two biomechanical wrenches into your body's movement patterns: they restrict the natural movement of your foot, and interfere with the proper function of your arch.

Why do men's shoes have heels?

One theory is that men's shoes have heels because they were designed to keep our feet in the stirrups while riding horses. Thousands of years ago, only the rich could afford horses, and they wore heeled footwear to ride. These shoes became a status symbol, even among those who couldn't afford a horse. Fast-forward through the centuries, and here we are today, unnaturally pitched forward as we go about our daily business.

The design of modern shoes, including running shoes, is not based on good science. [PAPER9]

What about those toe shoes that look like foot gloves? Do they simulate barefoot running, or help transition to barefoot running?

Of the few foot-glove runners I know, at least two have suffered stress fractures: (1) my cousin, a high school cross country runner; and (2) my next door neighbor, a former Division I college runner. I have to make myself scarce when their moms are in town, since I'm held responsible for introducing "barefoot running" into their lives.

When learning good form, your feet need to receive clear, unfiltered feedback from the ground. Every shoe interferes with that feedback, no matter what the ads say. [ARTICLE1]

Aren't you being a little rigid?

No. If you already have good running form, which often means you grew up running barefoot, you can wear minimalist shoes to protect your skin while running on rough trails. But you will have a difficult time *learning* good form without allowing your feet to feel the ground.

A recent article in the running press suggests that elite American runners are just as physically fit as the top Kenyans and Ethiopians, but lose on race day because the Africans have better form.

Form is everything – for performance, and more important, for long-term health.

My dad is 70-years-old, and he runs in his Nikes every morning. I can't accept that shoes are the problem.

Good for your dad, but what you've described is a classic example of "survivor bias."

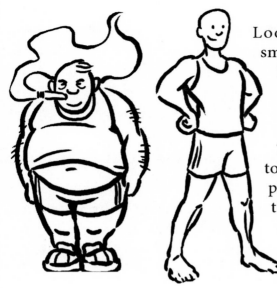

Look. We agree that smoking is bad for your health, right? If I'm the ad agency for a cigarette maker, could I find enough healthy 70-year-old smokers to put together a group photo op? With enough time and money, of course. Does that prove smoking is healthy? Of course not. To accurately measure the effect of smoking on health, we need to start with a large group of 20-year-old smokers and see how they fare over the next 50 years, relative to a similar group of non-smokers.

Running shod is a bit like that. Most one-time runners drop out over the decades of adulthood, because their "knees hurt" or their "back hurts." I want to yell at them, "It's not your knees or your back! It's your shoes!" The ones still running are the survivors. And they may not realize it, but they're the minority.

You are injured. That should tell you that your body is different from your dad's, and that you cannot follow in his shod running footsteps.

But I can wear them if I want, right? Let's say I want the benefits of running without restrictive shoes, but still want protection for my skin. No harm done?

Your feet don't need protection. When you are first learning to run with good form, the sensitivity of your skin is an asset, not a liability – it prevents you from doing too much too soon.

Only *when you are sure that you have mastered good running form*, if you want to try running on rough terrain, you might consider wearing minimalist shoes. At that point, look for shoes that don't have a raised heel, don't raise the toes, have a minimal sole with no arch support, and don't constrict your forefoot.

Is there any foot protection that simulates the benefits of barefoot running?

While learning to run with good form, your best option is to run barefoot whenever possible. Any footwear interferes with the feedback your body receives from the ground.

Unless the terrain is very rough, or the weather truly extreme, the risk of injury from running barefoot is very small.

What about those Masai shoes that look like rocking chairs?

My friends Justin and Laura visited Tanzania recently, and report that they did not see a single Masai wearing elevated rocking shoes.

Any shoe that raises you several inches above the ground greatly increases the danger of rolling an ankle. And that's exactly what happened to a friend who slipped while wearing these "rocking shoes" – she rolled sideways over her ankle, transmitting all the force of her falling body to her knee. She ended up with a "bucket handle meniscus tear," was in severe pain, needed a major surgery, and was on crutches for her leg as she sat at work, circulating ice water around her knee.

You do not want this to happen to you.

Avoid big raised soles.

How are shoe companies reacting to the increasing popularity of barefoot running?

Shoe companies and shoe retailers split into two groups: those who use fear to keep customers in their stinky shoes, and those who try to redefine the word "barefoot" to mean "running in our expensive brand-name shoes."

I admire the marketing savvy of the second group, but I have no reason to wear their shoes, and unless you are running in extreme conditions, neither do you. If your surroundings absolutely require shoes, there's considerable evidence that inexpensive shoes serve just as well, if not better. [PAPER5] [ARTICLE3]

Do shoes make you run faster or slower?

Shoes are weights moving at the end of a pendulum— your lower legs. The end is the "heaviest" position for a moving weight, requiring much more effort from you than another few ounces on your mid-section would. This is the same reason that bicyclists spend so much money buying extra light rims for their wheels.

Daniel Lieberman's barefoot running page [ARTICLE4] cites two research papers showing that barefoot runners use roughly 5% less energy. Losing the shoes should speed you up. Indeed, that's been my experience.

I encourage you to focus on running healthy, and let the speed develop when it will. Even a 15-minute/mile pace is so much faster and healthier than the "my knee hurts" couch potato alternative.

I insist on wearing Five Fingers some of the time. But they can get pretty stinky. How should I handle that?

The smell is caused by bacteria. My experience with other brands of rubbery sandals is that soaking them in a very weak bleach solution kills the bacteria and eliminates the smell. Rinse them off with water before wearing.

I can't believe I just aided and abetted the wearing of those hideous shoes!

How about racing flats?

Most Americans did not grow up running barefoot, and do not have perfect form. To learn form, we are better off running barefoot (skin to ground).

Racing flats and other minimalist shoes often cause injuries when worn by non-expert runners with less than excellent form.

Once you're a full-fledged barefoot runner, is wearing shoes in other circumstances uncomfortable? Barefoot business meetings are not common!

Most of us must wear shoes in daily life. Look for shoes that do not constrict or "support" your feet.

Why are you approving minimalist shoes for work when you don't like them for running?

Walking causes less impact than running, so even with imperfect form, you're less likely to hurt yourself when wearing minimalist shoes. When walking, as when running, be sure to lift your feet rather than push off.

How important is heel drop?

You want a shoe with no raised heel. Why? Because your arch requires level supports at both ends. That's how we were born and how the human body evolved to move.

By the same token, I do not recommend negative heel shoes. The best way to run is the way we were designed to run – without foot-constraining or modifying devices.

I read in *Born to Run* that the Tarahumara tribe in Mexico run long distances wearing Huarache rope sandals. If they don't run barefoot, why should I?

The Tarahumara, like elite Kenyan and Ethiopian runners, learn excellent running form by spending much of their childhood going barefoot. Once you have good form, if you need to run on rugged terrain, it's a good idea to wear protection against sharp rocks.

How should the novice barefoot runner navigate rocky terrain?

For at least your first six months running barefoot, I suggest staying on paved roads. Think of it as an investment in a lifetime of health. If you absolutely must run a rocky trail, wear minimalist running shoes without a raised heel.

Humans have been wearing protective shoes for as long as they could wrap their feet in hides and vegetation – before advertising. They must have had a reason. Why change now?

Humans wrapped their feet in animal hide when conditions required it, as when they moved from Africa to the cold climates of Northern Europe.

Wrapping your feet in hide to protect them from sharp rocks or extreme temperatures is one thing. Wearing heavy shoes with rigid arch supports and high cushioned heels is another.

I like my high heels!

Research suggests that long-term use of high-heeled shoes damages women's feet and their backs. It also leads to shorter muscles and thickened, stiffened Achilles tendons. [PAPER11] [PAPER17]

I hate to separate a girl from her Manolo Blahniks, but why not limit your Manolo binges to special occasions, and then wear flats for routine walking?

On a related note, I just got this email from a friend:

> "I was having crazy joint pain when I was wearing heels AND dancing, which I have completely eradicated not by stopping dancing (which I thought was the problem) but by not wearing heels. I invested in some cute flats too. :-)
>
> Suggest trying no heels for a couple of weeks to see how it feels (amazing)."

Some people would kill for a cool, fashionable pair of shoes. They're a status symbol. Do you really think people will give this up to look like third-world paupers?

That's a key issue: how much function (injury-free running and good health) are you willing to sacrifice to look good? Some people will choose health, others fashion. Either is a legitimate choice if it's made with full knowledge of the facts.

I received a mailer from a major shoe retailer that called barefoot running "Maximum Nonsense," and warned of the "pea-size rocks just waiting to take a big bite out of [my] feet."

Sadly, I don't have such creative ad writers in my camp! All I have is the facts.

I leave it to you to balance the shoe industry's rhetoric with the research presented here, as well as the feedback from your own two feet. Decide for yourself. Don't let anyone scare you. Don't let anyone decide for you.

If barefoot running is so much better and more natural, then why does the running shoe industry continue to boom, designing and re-designing their products? Shouldn't we have reverted to our primitive ways by now?

Consider how long we've had cigarettes. Bad-for-you products can thrive, as long as there's something to advertise and sell.

Running shoes are a multi-billion dollar industry, with big marketing budgets and a strong sense of self-preservation.

The modern running shoe was born around 1970. Forty years isn't a long lifespan for a bad idea, especially for one that's so profitable.

Running shoes feel good. Why should I change?

You might consider the damage caused to your wallet and to the environment, but if it's working for you, I don't really expect you to change. That's why this book is aimed at runners over the age of 30, which is when soreness no longer disappears overnight, and we become more motivated to treat our bodies well.

Then again, if you do try a few minutes of barefoot running, you may find that it's actually … fun.

What should I do with my old running shoes? Should I send them to Africa?

No. Like Americans, Africans are better off running barefoot. Nike's Reuse-A-Shoe program is one of many that recycles the rubber from old shoes.

What shoes do you wear when not running?

When the situation requires wearing shoes, which is most of the time when I'm going somewhere, I wear minimal footwear – minimal soles, minimal binding around the forefoot and no raised heel. Whenever possible, I wear two-dollar flip-flops, also known as thongs.

For women, flats are preferable to heels. But you knew that.

In the U.S., it is surprisingly difficult to find formal men's shoes without a raised heel. Perhaps men's flats will catch on as the disadvantages of heels become better known.

[**Summary:**   Shoes damage your feet.]

But My Doctor Says ...

But my doctor says that runners need to have good shoes. Why aren't the experts convinced that barefoot running is better?

Keep in mind that most MDs are not researchers. They have a lot on their mind, and are not in fact experts on footwear choice. I'm sure your doctor means well, but many doctors are only quoting what they were taught about feet in medical school, often decades ago.

Scientific evidence strongly favors running barefoot or in minimal shoes that protect against the elements but do not "support" the foot. There is no evidence that "supportive" shoes do any good, while there *is* evidence that they do harm. [PAPER9] [PAPER11] [PAPER12]

Has this topic been studied by scientists?

Yes, extensively. The more I look into it, the more I am surprised by the amount of research pointing in the same direction, yet under the radar of many physicians. Perhaps the benefits of barefooting will be taught in medical schools in the next decade, which means that doctors 20 or 30 years from now will have their facts straight.

Is barefoot running the best option for everybody, or should I get an opinion from an orthopedist?

Always consult your physician before beginning a new exercise regimen, even more so if you have a unique or especially challenging condition. Diabetes, hemophilia, Charcot-Marie-Tooth disease, and any peripheral neuropathy are conditions that may suggest against running barefoot.

I donate blood regularly. Can I still run barefoot? I heard that the impact of running can lower my iron levels (footstrike hemolysis).

I give blood every eight weeks, and my iron levels are fine. When you run barefoot, your body adjusts its form so that the impact force may actually be less than when you wear shoes.

If you are concerned about anemia, have your hemoglobin levels checked. Also, consider using iron cookware. It's inexpensive, replenishes your iron levels and reduces the amount of potentially toxic anti-stick coating in your food. Besides, an iron skillet just looks cool.

Why does my podiatrist recommend against barefoot running?

Podiatrists, like MDs, don't perform a research study for each patient. They apply whatever they were told in podiatry school.

To some extent, we are responsible for our own health these days. Read my interviews with two well-regarded podiatrists who have given a great deal of thought to the topic of barefoot running, read the research presented in the next chapter, talk to other barefoot runners, and consider politely asking your podiatrist for his or her reasoning.

Some podiatrists, though not all, believe in the paradigm that the human body is inherently weak and therefore we need big shoes and orthotics to compensate for the shortcomings of the foot.

That's one point of view. Another view is that barring disuse or misuse, the human body is great at most things, if technology would just get out of the way. We don't need to be "fixed" to move around.

What are the other health effects of barefoot running?

Moving from science to the anecdotal realm, many runners report better health while running barefoot. For instance, I've had only one cold in the almost three years that I've been running barefoot. My only explanation is that it might have something to do with stimulating reflexology points on the foot. Reflexology has only been lightly researched in the West, but check out [PAPER15].

What are the best painkillers to use for barefoot running?

You should never, ever, run while taking painkillers. You can seriously injure your legs by running through pain that is signaling you to stop, and you could severely and permanently damage your kidneys.

The point of barefoot running is to reduce pain and injuries. Slight soreness may indicate that your body is adapting, but anything more than that warns of a problem that needs to be addressed. Fix the problem; don't cover up the symptoms. You should not require painkillers – even after a run.

Twice in my running career I've used strong painkillers prescribed by doctors for injuries that I now realize were caused by poor running form exacerbated by running shoes. These problems have not recurred since I took off the shoes, even as I run farther and faster.

I know that the medical system is looking out for my health. Why should I trust what you tell me?

Well, don't take my word for it. Read the interviews, and read the science.

And let's look at some of my running injury-related medical visits and the associated costs. I list the total cost, most of it borne by insurance:

BEFORE BAREFOOT:

- ▶ Two or three pairs of orthotics: $200-$300 each.
- ▶ One MRI, for what turned out to be ITBS: around $1,000.
- ▶ Twenty or more deep-tissue massage treatments for ITBS: around $80 each.
- ▶ Corns removed (twice): $500 per treatment. Apparently, it's a "surgical procedure."
- ▶ Twenty or more sessions of physical therapy for ITBS and Achilles tendonitis: $100-$250 per session.
- ▶ Several visits to orthopedists and podiatrists: $150 per visit.
- ▶ Cortisone injection for plantar fasciitis: $200.

AFTER BAREFOOT:

- ▶ In the nearly three years (and two marathons) since I began running barefoot, my legs have required no medical attention at all, so my health insurers and I have paid $0 to podiatrists, orthopedists, physical therapists, orthotics manufacturers and other medical professionals and suppliers. As you read the interviews, and talk to barefoot runners in your own community, you'll learn that my story is the rule, rather than the exception.

Which of the scenarios above is more beneficial for the medical industry? Which is more beneficial for patients like you and me – not to mention our healthcare system as a whole?

Make your own decision, but do it with full knowledge of the facts.

Summary: Modern medical care is a good thing. So is informing yourself with the facts and asking your doctor a lot of questions.

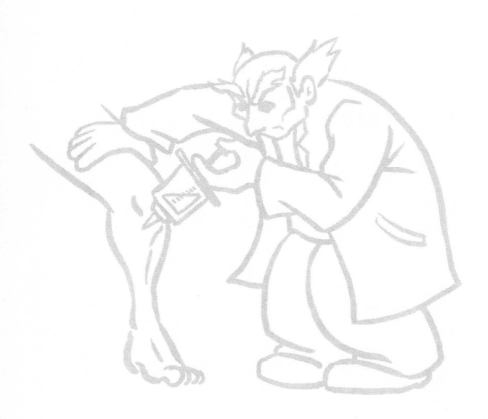

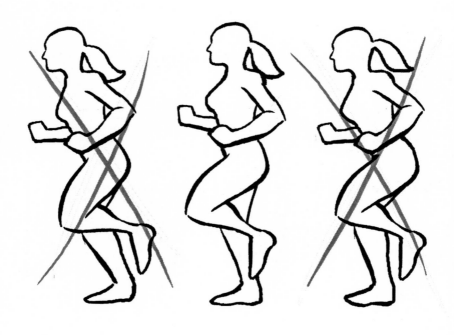

Remember: Keep Your Hips Forward

Interview:

Meet The Podiatrist:
Dr. Michael Nirenberg

And you are ...?

Dr. Michael Nirenberg. I am a doctor of podiatric medicine, and a podiatric surgeon, practicing in Crown Point, Indiana. I am also a forensic podiatrist, meaning I am one of the handful of forensic podiatrists in the world who assist law enforcement in analyzing footwear and foot prints and foot-related evidence at crime scenes.

Forensic podiatrist? Like ... CSI?

Dr. Nirenberg: Yeah, feet are remarkable. They can reveal a lot about the body.

So, doctor, now that we live in the 21st century, why would somebody want to go barefoot?

Dr. Nirenberg: For most people who are in good health, I believe that walking barefoot, when you are in a safe area, is healthier than wearing shoes.

Anthropologists tell us that for about 3.6 million years, at least, we've walked upright on two feet. For the vast majority of that time we walked and we ran barefoot or with flimsy moccasin-like sandals. It is only in the last several hundred years that we started wearing footwear, and there are changes to our feet as a result of wearing footwear.

It's well documented that footwear, most of the time, is harmful and detrimental to our feet.

On the simplest level, if your shoe has the lowest of arches, if your running shoe is even an inch off the ground at the heel, or three quarters of an inch, you are allowing your foot to sit on a bit of an angle, your heel is high and your toes are low, and what this does is, it creates an imbalance between the muscles on the top of your foot and your muscles on the bottom.

On top of that, most of these shoes that we use for walking and running now pride themselves on being supportive, and the more you use support, the more your muscles do not have to work. We have four layers of muscles in the bottom of our foot, and we have muscles from our leg entering our foot. Most of these muscles do not have to work in supportive shoes. Like the old saying goes, "Use it or lose it."

If you lose that muscle strength in your foot, then when you are not in a supportive shoe one day, or you stress your foot excessively with activity or exercise, suddenly, abruptly, the muscles are not prepared, and they are not strong enough to provide the support you need. Then the support falls to your ligaments and soft tissue structure, and you're at risk for injury.

Most people solve this by buying arch support. You know, in the short term, arch support is good at alleviating pain. But in the long term, the more you use it, the more you become dependent, or in one manner of speaking, your foot may become physiologically addicted to support.

Running shoes are a multi-billion-dollar industry. How could running shoes have succeeded without providing any benefit?

Dr. Nirenberg: I am not so sure how we got here. There have been people warning of the hazards of shoes through the '20s, '30s, '40s and '50s. Books were published by people warning of the hazards of shoes, but the message has gotten drowned out.

Most people do not have a lot of confidence and faith in their own two feet. They have bought into the advertising – into the need for support.

But the truth is, feet are incredibly resilient. They can take a lot of abuse. They manage to walk, and carry the body forward, and balance and get through 80 years or more, walking miles everyday.

Some podiatrists echo your sentiments about the resilience of feet, and others disagree. Why is that?

Dr. Nirenberg: These doctors have gone to podiatry school, where they were taught that feet need good support – orthotics, arch support. You are asking people who have been doing this for many years to re-think everything that they've learned.

It is hard to change a mindset. For millions of years, people thought the world was flat, and people thought that the earth was the center of the universe. You know, people [once] thought that formula was the best thing for babies. Now, they realize it is breast milk.

So, these doctors are well intentioned, they want to do the right thing, and yet some of them are incapable of opening their minds to it.

Thanks for your insights, Dr. Nirenberg. How can injured runners get in touch with you?

Dr. Nirenberg: Through my website www.AmericasPodiatrist. com.

Summary: The muscles in your feet - use it or lose it.

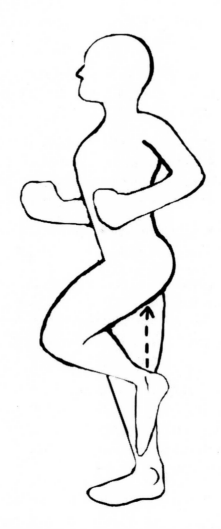

***

Remember: Don't Push Off

What Does Science Prove About Barefoot Running?

What does science prove about barefoot running?

The existing scientific evidence strongly suggests that we're better off without built-up shoes. Forty years after running shoes became all the rage, there isn't one shred of scientific evidence to support the use of these shoes. [PAPER9]

Health claims are regulated by the government. So if shoe companies say running shoes work, it must be true.

You would think so. Pharmaceuticals need to go through years of testing to gain FDA approval, and then any health claims made on their behalf are closely regulated. In contrast, multi-billion-dollar running shoe companies are apparently free to advertise whatever benefits their marketing department dreams up, with nary a check or balance.

It all reminds me of Coca Cola's advertising campaign for its Vitaminwater drinks. In defending against a recent lawsuit alleging that Coke made false health claims on behalf of Vitaminwater, the company responded (according to the judge's report) that "no consumer could reasonably be misled into thinking Vitaminwater was a healthy beverage." [ARTICLE7]

It makes me wonder, is that also the running shoe companies' defense to all the evidence in favor of barefoot running: that no consumer could believe their advertising?

What evidence shows that barefoot running is better?

What evidence shows that running in $130 shoes is better? I'll tell you: none. See the study titled, "Is Your Prescription of Distance Running Shoes Evidence Based?" [PAPER9]

Since we didn't enter life wearing heavy, expensive, heel-raised sneakers, isn't the burden of proof on the shoe pushers?

The US Military commissioned three large studies (Army, Air Force, Marines) to reduce injuries among exercising soldiers by improving their running shoe choice.

"We found no scientific basis for choosing running shoes based on foot type," said Bruce Jones, M.D., injury prevention program manager at U.S. Army Public Health Command (Provisional), Aberdeen Proving Ground, Maryland. "Our findings have surprised not just military decision-makers – many of whom run to stay fit – but runners in general."

Popular running and sports medicine literature recommends that people with high arches should choose **cushioning shoes**, those with normal arches should choose **stability shoes**, and those with flat feet should choose **motion-control shoes**, Jones explained. The literature says that such shoes will compensate for the way these foot types strike the ground during running and lessen injuries to the legs and feet.

"This seemed to many of us to make sense," said Jones, a long-distance runner for many years. "But when we looked at it in multiple, scientific studies, it turned out to be a **sports myth.**" [ARTICLE6]

"Sports myth!" Ouch.

So the military, hardly a tree-hugging organization, finds that what "everyone knows" about running shoes, and what every running shoe salesperson tells you, is a myth. Will they take the logical next step of considering barefoot running (during peacetime)? I hope so.

A good friend of mine owns a running shoe store, and writes a column on running. He thinks barefoot running is a fad based on pseudo-science. How would you respond to him?

Running shoes are a multi-billion dollar industry, and yet there's not one single study showing the efficacy of running shoes in preventing injury. On the contrary, many studies suggest that shoes increase forces on the legs and aggravate injuries, and plenty of anecdotal evidence suggests the same.

We evolved to run barefoot. Which one is the fad – bare feet, or shoes? [PAPER4] [PAPER9] [PAPER12] [PAPER13] [PAPER14]

I know how strong the emotional tie to running shoes can be – I was the same way for many years. If your friend is wedded to the idea that we must have something on our feet, facts are unlikely to change his mind. But the next time he's laid up with a running injury, I think you know what to give him for convalescent light reading.

Which cultures today are shoeless, and how are they doing with the barefoot thing?

Few cultures today are completely shoeless, but unshod cultures have historically had a much lower incidence of foot and lower leg injuries. [PAPER3] [PAPER14]

Recent research suggests that shoes were invented about 30,000 years ago. Simple foot coverings make sense to protect the feet against harsh conditions. It's the evolution of shoes from "protection against the elements" to "assistive device" that has caused unintended and harmful consequences. [PAPER2] [PAPER6]

Can I still enjoy some benefits if I only run barefoot half the time?

Barefoot running is easier on your body, and it will help you develop good form you can use when wearing shoes. Over time, you might want to limit your use of heel-lifted shoes, including built-up running shoes. Better yet, eliminate those shoes from your wardrobe.

Summary: Much scientific evidence supports barefooting. No evidence supports built-up running shoes.

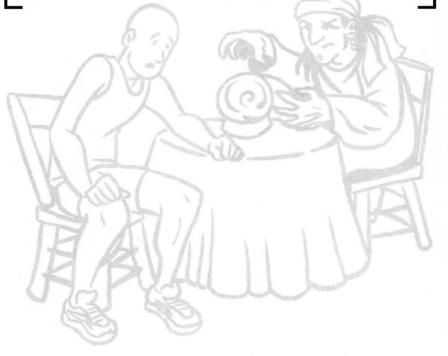

Interview:

Cassie Howard:
"[My Shoes Hurt] ... So I Ran Home Barefoot"

And you are ...?

My name is *Cassie Howard.* I am 31, and live in the Chicago suburbs. It's a small town – Elgin, Illinois. I'm a stay-at-home mom. I have a three-year-old and a one-year-old, and they keep me busy. My life revolves around them during the day.

What's your running history?

Cassie: I am new to running. I started in July [2010], with one of those couch-to-5K programs. I started out slow, running with whatever cheap shoes I had in my house. Then I hit the fifth week – a 20-minute run.

It's the first time I ran for any length of time, and I hurt. My knees hurt, my hips hurt and my ankles hurt. I wanted to cry.

I went on the *Runner's World* website, and they said to go to a local running store and get real running shoes. I went to the store, and I was expecting this wonderful experience— you know, they analyzed my gait and everything. I came home with a great pair of shoes, or so I thought. The next morning, I put them on and went for a run, and my feet went numb from about the middle of my arch downward. I thought, "Oh, maybe I laced them wrong. They are too tight." So I loosened them and kept going, but my feet were still numb … dead. There was no feeling at all.

I took the shoes off. I was about a mile from home, so I ran home barefoot. I really fell into it by accident. It still tickles me. But at the time, I thought, "I need new shoes," so I took my shoes back to the store. I ended up doing that two more times, going through three pairs of shoes. Finally, they said, "You've tried every pair of shoes in the store. We can't help you. You need to see a doctor." I thought, "I don't need to see a doctor. Not if I can run barefoot." Then, I started doing my research.

Now, [running barefoot] I don't hurt anywhere – my feet, my ankles, my knees, my hips – so yeah, I fell into it and it's been wonderful.

It took me years of disbelief and research before I was brave enough to run barefoot. And you just did it.

Cassie: I didn't know any better, because I was a new runner. I didn't know I shouldn't take off my shoes and run, or I might get injuries from too much, too soon.

How was the transition to going barefoot?

Cassie: Wonderful. Today, I'm up to about six mile barefoot runs. I've been home for three years, not wearing shoes, so I've progressed quickly.

What do your friends and neighbors have to say?

Cassie: A lot of them are stuck on the social stigma. They don't want to be seen as "lower class." It's like "poor people don't wear shoes."

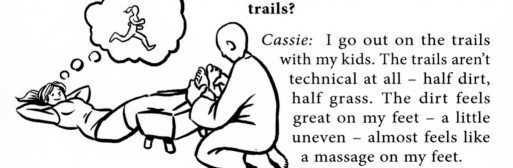

Where do you run? Do you run on trails?

Cassie: I go out on the trails with my kids. The trails aren't technical at all – half dirt, half grass. The dirt feels great on my feet – a little uneven – almost feels like a massage on my feet.

Any advice for beginners?

Cassie: Listen to your own body.

All these how-to guides say: "Go slow. Walk in place for a day." That was too slow for me. They tell you, "Lift your knees, do this, do that," and I'm trying to run and think about these things all at once. It was too much. It was overwhelming me, and I would get aches and pains. I was concentrating on what somebody else told me, and wasn't doing what felt best. Finally, I stopped reading so much, and went with myself. And it was so much better.

After our conversation, Cassie wrote to say:

Cassie: After the birth of my youngest son, I started to experience pain in my back and leg – down into my foot. I saw physical therapists, chiropractors and an orthopedic surgeon. It turns out that I had two herniated disks in my lower back. I could not sit, lie down or walk without pain.

I had two steroid injections to help with the inflammation, but it wasn't until I began running barefoot that I started healing. I increased my blood flow, and the barefoot running helped my body with alignment. During the first year after my son's birth, I was in pain 98% of the time. I'm still not 100%, but the only time I experience back pain is when I lie down, and it's more of an annoyance than real pain.

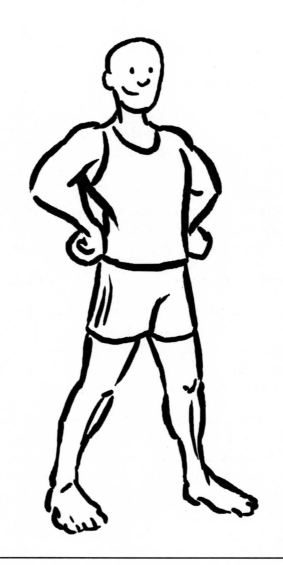

Remember: Stand Tall

Why Doesn't Haile Run Barefoot?

Why doesn't marathon world record holder Haile Gebrselassie run barefoot?

As a child, Gebrselassie grew up barefoot, running several miles to and from school every day, so his good running form is ingrained. These days, he's paid a lot of money to endorse shoes, so that's what he does – and indeed, he is often injured.

At any open track meet, you will notice that most of the top non-collegiate runners are sponsored by shoe companies. Might be tough for a barefoot runner to find a sponsor.

Maybe runners who exceed 100 miles/week, month after month (especially at the pace these guys run), do need minimal foot covering to protect their skin from abrading. Note that elite African runners do not wear the built-up shoes that you and I are sold. They wear the lightest possible racing shoe, to displays the sponsor's brand while not interfering with their naturally good form.

Last but not least, what young athletes do to achieve peak performance may not be the best foundation for long-term health. Just take a look at baseball, NFL Football, and professional bicycling.

If African runners switch to shoes as soon as they can afford them, that's hardly a ringing endorsement of going barefoot.

As I was saying, many African runners grow up running barefoot, for fun, in an unstructured way. This is when they develop their impeccable running form. The best of them compete barefoot at the top levels of junior running. Then, at the age of 16 or 17, when they are ready to move to the senior league, they join running camps, all sponsored by shoe companies, where they are required to compete in shoes.

In addition to the Africans who grew up running without shoes, many top Western runners also include barefoot running as a part of their training program.

Have any barefoot runners won races?

The most famous barefoot running performance of all time is probably Abebe Bikila's win at the 1960 Rome Olympics Marathon – the first-ever gold medal for a black African runner.

In the 1980s, Zola Budd held the world record for the women's 5,000 meters, running barefoot. Also barefoot, she twice won the Women's World Cross Country Championships.

Zola Budd didn't do so well at the '84 Olympics, as I recall. Is that a warning to the rest of us?

In the final of the 3,000 meters at the 1984 Olympic Games, Mary Decker collided with Zola Budd and then (Decker) tumbled to the ground. The collision was not Budd's fault, much less the fault of Budd's bare feet.

Who else?

Other barefoot champions:

- ▶ Bruce Tulloh set several European records in the 1950s and 1960s while running barefoot.
- ▶ Shivnath Singh holds the barefoot marathon record of 2 hours and 12 minutes, at a faster pace than most of us can dream of running even one mile. As in Africa, many Indian runners go barefoot because they cannot afford running shoes. They may not realize that they actually have an advantage!
- ▶ Charlie "Doc" Robbins was a physician who won several U.S. middle-distance championships running barefoot.
- ▶ Michelle Dekkers won the 1988 NCAA cross country championships running barefoot.
- ▶ In Feb 2011, Dejen Gebremeskel won the 3,000 meters at the New Balance Indoor Grand Prix wearing just one shoe, after losing the other one at the start. Makes you wonder why the others bothered with their track spikes. [VIDEO6]

The list goes on. In many parts of the world, from Africa to India to New Zealand, running barefoot is commonplace, so barefoot victories aren't always highlighted in the record books.

Most of us will never win a race, but each of us can maintain a healthy running routine well into old age.

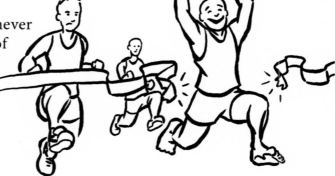

Would I be able to compete against shod runners if I run barefoot, or would I be at a considerable disadvantage?

If injuries are holding you back, there's a good chance that barefoot running will allow you to increase your training load and, therefore, run faster. If you are a mid-pack marathoner, losing the shoes will not immediately move you into the ranks of top Americans Ryan Hall and Meb Keflezighi.

Have you been able to beat your performance while shod?

Yes. After more than 20 years of running, my best times over every distance are while running barefoot, and I continue to improve even as I age.

The improvement may partly be due to the absence of shoes weighing down my feet during a race, and partly because I can run many more miles in training, without injury, than I ever could when shod.

Are extreme long-distance runners doing this?

In the U.S., a small but growing number of marathoners compete barefoot. A few barefoot ultra-marathoners also run races of over 50 miles.

Summary: Run barefoot for good health. Winning races may or may not follow.

Interview:

Julian Romero: "I'll Show You My Feet If You Promise To Touch Them"

And you are ...?

I'm *Julian Romero*. I'm 27, I have a PhD from Caltech, and recently began a new job as a professor at Purdue. [VIDEO3]

Tell us about your running history.

Julian: I went to Albuquerque High School, where I ran cross country, and then to Northwestern University, where I played baseball. I was always lifting weights, and that's why I'm a bit heavier than most runners.

And were you always a barefoot runner?

Julian: No. I think if you run cross country in high school, you just develop a love for running. So, after my baseball career ended on graduating from Northwestern, I was very excited to start running again. I started running in shoes in the summer of 2005.

My younger brother (2:40 marathoner Alex Romero) had been telling me about how barefoot running was good. He had an excellent high school cross country career, and when he got to college, he was running in the biggest, most padded shoes he could find, and he just struggled his entire college career with injuries. Barefoot running really turned things around for him.

So, I decided to give it a try after running the San Francisco Marathon. One thing that I loved about running barefoot was, six steps into my run, I immediately knew what I was doing wrong. So, I did that run – I think it was a four- or five-mile run – thinking, "This feels pretty good, but I probably won't jump into it right away."

The next day, I was planning on running half barefoot, half shoes. I'd found this really nice trail in Pasadena. So, I took my shoes out there, and went running. I did a 10-mile run or something, and my feet just felt horrible. I think it was because I'd done my first barefoot run the day before, and my feet were sore. But just having those tight shoes pressing all around my feet – it felt like the shoes were really making my feet hurt. At that point, I thought, "I've had enough of this. I'm going to give this barefoot running thing a try." I haven't run in typical running shoes since that 10-miler.

What about arch support? Don't you need arch support?

Julian: When people ask me about arch support, the analogy I like to use is this: Let's say you sprain your ankle, and you go to the doctor. The doctor says, "Your ankle looks like you sprained it pretty bad. How about you walk on crutches for a week? Come back and see me after a week." So, you walk around on your crutches for a week, and then go back. The doctor says, "Looks like your sprain is a bit better, but your ankle still looks pretty weak. How about you walk on crutches for another week?" So, you walk on crutches for another week, and go back again. Now, the doctor says, "Your ankle doesn't look any stronger. In fact, it looks like it's getting weaker, so how about using a wheelchair for next week?"

If you never use the muscle, it's never going to get strong. If you have a weak arch, and you support it with arch supports or orthotics, it's just going to get weaker, which means you'll have to do even *more* to support the muscle.

The alternative is to try to strengthen it. An arch is one of the most amazing physical structures that bears weight. It just doesn't make sense to support an arch from the bottom when you can strengthen it and use the strength of the arch.

What else do you enjoy about barefoot running?

Julian: You don't have to buy shoes. I have really big feet, so packing a size 13 pair of running shoes gets heavy. When running barefoot, you don't have to pack anything.

That helps, especially with all the carry-on restrictions.

Julian: There was a documentary from the Canadian Broadcasting Company that had (barefoot runner) Ken Bob in it. They did something on the marathon. They had Ken Bob and this other lady, who brought like seven pairs of running shoes to the Las Vegas Marathon. That would be so annoying.

It's also really nice to be able to just feel the different surfaces. I live next to the Wabash River, where there are some really nice trails with almost no rocks. There are quite a few sticks, and it's really muddy, but it's really nice to go out on a hot summer afternoon and feel the cool mud under your feet.

Also, I really love running when it's hot. If you go out when it's 100 degrees, and run on the hot pavement, when you come back you feel like you have warm cookies on your feet.

On a hot day, like the day of the (2010) Chicago Marathon, it's really nice because you don't have to have your feet trapped inside socks and shoes. You can feel the breeze on your feet, which keeps you cool.

What are some favorite comments that you've heard?

Julian: I heard a good one during the Chicago Marathon. As I was running by, this guy said, "Hey look. There's a barefoot runner." He was saying this to a friend. "He's going to put you out of business." I don't know what his friend did, but I guess he was a podiatrist or owns a shoe store. I looked over at his friend, and he was wearing two knee bands for pain.

Love it!

Julian: It was pretty funny.

I think it's funny when people get mad at you. They act like they are experts. They say "you are so stupid," or that you shouldn't be doing what you're doing.

One time, a guy stopped his car, and literally put his entire torso out the window to yell at me, telling me how stupid I was to run barefoot. I found it interesting that somebody would get so angry over that.

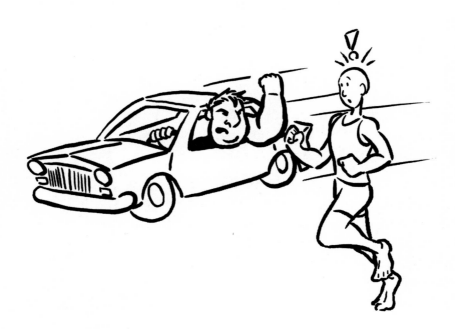

Where Can I Run?

Where can I run? Is barefoot running safe in an urban environment?

For the most part, yes. That's where I run.

I see occasional broken glass on my regular routes, and I get a splinter about every six months. If I felt I was running through broken glass every day, I'd probably choose another route.

Running barefoot *does* require that you be aware of your surroundings, which is good practice for all runners.

Indoors on a treadmill?

If you must. We weren't really designed to run with the ground moving under us, but I understand that weather and safety considerations may occasionally send us to the treadmill.

Do gyms allow barefoot running?

Unfortunately, many gyms do not allow barefoot running, because they misunderstand existing local health codes, or claim "liability." If health codes required shoes, the prisons would be full of swim coaches and yoga teachers.

Gyms exist to serve their patrons. Arm yourself with the facts, and let the management know that you prefer to run barefoot. If enough barefoot runners state their needs, the rules will be changed, since there is no good reason to require shoes.

Barefoot running on a glass-free, clutter-free beach is safe. I'm not sure where else you can run without encountering a sprinkler head, dog poop, glass or some other object.

The world is not as dangerous as you fear. Once in a while you will step on something unpleasant, but in my experience, injuries from sharp debris are fewer and less severe than the impact injuries from shod running.

Beaches are fun, but turn out to be not that good for long runs, because of the slope as well as abrasion from the sand.

I've never stepped in dog poop on a run. I did step in some at my investment banker friend's backyard BBQ. And I lived to tell the tale.

A bird has pooped on me, but a shoe wouldn't have helped, as it quickly flew out of shoe-throwing range. My point is: poop happens. It's unpleasant, but it's a minor annoyance without long-term consequences.

Isn't it extremely hot to run barefoot on the street during the summer?

Yes. Midday, midsummer asphalt can be painful, though you do build up tolerance over time. On really hot days, I often run on the painted white lines. A better solution during the hottest days of summer is to run in the morning.

How much does the surface that you run on matter?

Most hard surfaces that are not strewn with obvious hazards will be fine.

Running on roads seems too scary. I think I'll stick to grass.

Running on hard surfaces lets you use feedback from your feet to learn good, efficient form. Grass is soft, and allows you to run any old way, with very bad form. In addition, grass can hide divots, broken glass and other nasties.

In short, running on grass, though superficially attractive, doesn't help you learn, and may do more harm than good.

Likewise, artificial turf is too soft to provide the feedback you need to develop good form, and unlike grass, it can get extremely hot in the sun.

So what are the very best places to run barefoot?

The best starting place is a clean and smooth road or sidewalk. Once you have at least six months experience, begin to experiment with trails. At that point, feel free to run wherever you most enjoy it.

As your feet regain their natural strength, you might try increasingly rugged trails. Even after years of barefoot running, you will always be able to find new challenges in new surfaces. More yummy feedback for your feet.

What about running on chipseal?

Chipseal is a very rough pavement surface, common in rural areas. As with any harsh surface, this can be hard on the beginning barefoot runner. On the plus side, running on chipseal will probably stop you from hurting yourself by doing too much too soon. Over time, your feet will become accustomed to it.

What about running in the winter?

I've run a marathon with the start temperature at 28 degrees. In Kansas City, "Barefoot Rick" runs in snow every winter.

If it's well below freezing, however, you may want to run indoors, or wear minimal shoes to prevent frostbite.

How early or late in the season do you recommend running barefoot?

In California, I run barefoot all year around, occasionally running on the white lines in mid-summer, or sliding across patches of ice in the winter. Where I live, it gets down to freezing, but not much below.

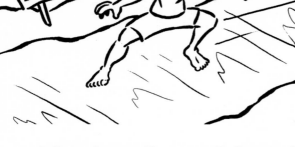

If I lived in Minnesota, I'd probably wear minimal shoes, or run indoors in the winter.

What about oil, gas and chemicals on the ground?

This was initially a concern for me. The consensus is that the risk in most areas is no more than the risk we face from chemicals in the industrialized environment all around us.

What about bacteria and viruses on the ground?

Asphalt is a harsh environment for viruses and bacteria, thanks to UV light and desiccation. In fact, the shopping cart you push around the grocery store with your bare hands is almost certainly more germ-ridden than the road.

In addition, human skin, in the absence of cuts, is a good barrier against most pathogens. Of course, if you are regularly putting your bare feet in your mouth, you'll want to wash them first.

If I'm going to run barefoot, what routes should I start with? I hate tracks and neighborhoods.

Run wherever you want to. Barefoot running is about having fewer rules and requirements instead of more. You don't need a particular shoe technology, and you don't need a particular route design or surface.

Isn't the ground hot or wet or uncomfortable?

Usually not, and your feet adapt. When you first start to run barefoot, hot or wet or rough surfaces may feel uncomfortable. This is actually a good thing, as it prevents you from doing too much, too soon.

What about running at night?

I prefer to run during the day, when I can see where I'm going. Some nighttime barefoot runners practice stepping very gently and "seeing" only with their feet. After dark, I recommend running only on paths that you know well, and using a lightweight LED flashlight or headlamp.

What about running barefoot in the military?

Several service members belong to online barefoot running forums. Military rules about bare feet seem to differ, depending on the service and the location.

First of all, of course, obey your orders. And any time you find yourself wearing body armor and a helmet, you'll want something on your feet, too.

Summary: You can run barefoot most places. Just use common sense.

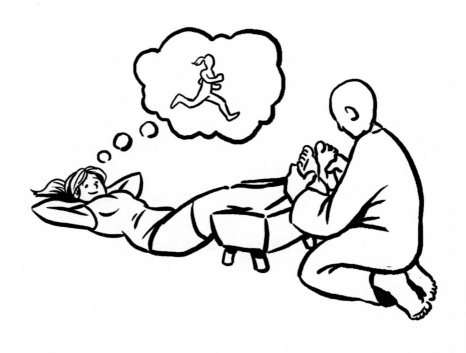

Remember: Relax

Interview:

Angie B: "If You're Not Having Fun, What's The Point?"

And you are ...?

Angie B, 33, married and the mother of four boys. I live in Des Moines, Iowa. I used to live in Kona, where the Ironman World Championship race is held, and I worked at a pizza place that was about a quarter mile from the start and finish of this triathlon. I got inspired, and decided to run a marathon. My first marathon was Honolulu in 1998.

So, you've been running for a while. How long barefoot?

Angie: When my fourth son was born, I felt this urge to start running again. I wanted to lose the baby weight and get thin again. So, I started learning about nutrition and how to change my eating habits, and running fell right into place with all that. I didn't have to go to a gym and worry about childcare.

I ran a couple of 5Ks, and I ran a 20K race called the "Dam to Dam," where you go up to the Saylorville Lake Reservoir Dam, and then run back to the city to another dam. I ran the race, and it just felt awful. I had horrible shin splits. I couldn't train very much for it, because my shins hurt so much.

After I had the kids, especially the last two, I noticed that my lower back was never quite the same. I would lean too far back and push my pelvis out. I had this very uncomfortable pinched nerve in my back. Wearing the running shoes with the raised heel would exaggerate that.

How did you know the raised heel was the problem?

Angie: I didn't at the time. All I knew was that it hurt. It was very frustrating. Still, I needed to run. I wanted alone time where I could meditate on the things that I needed to deal with. But I couldn't get enough miles in, because of my injuries. Then, my husband read an article online, and suggested that I ditch the shoes.

I thought, "You're crazy! You don't know what you're talking about. I have to have my shoes. I have to have stability."

This was around the end of May 2009, right when *Born to Run* came out. I read the book, and was so inspired that I apologized to my husband, saying, "Thanks for making me read this book and suggesting barefoot running." I was in love with the book. Even before I reached the end of it, I wanted to try. It was so inspiring.

Even after reading *Born to Run*, I didn't ditch my shoes completely. It took about two weeks of running. I would run barefoot for a quarter mile, and wear shoes for another quarter to half mile.

I'd run barefoot, and then put my shoes on, but as my barefoot running increased, I couldn't find that form. I couldn't find that feeling again when I put on my shoes. When I got to running about three miles barefoot, I decided to get rid of the shoes. I couldn't run in them any more. I just felt lost in them. I couldn't feel what I was doing.

I was enjoying barefoot running. It gave me a sense of purpose; it gave me goals. I was excited about it, and the limited amount of mileage I was able to do didn't matter. I wasn't upset about that.

Some people find it hard to drop the mileage down. But I looked at it this way: if I continued to learn how to run barefoot, then there would be [eventually] no limitations on how far I could run.

I know you run on a treadmill. Can you talk about that?

Angie: Some treadmills get really hot. Mine is really comfortable, but I know a couple of people who can't run more than a mile on the treadmill [because of the heat]. If that's an issue, then I would think that running with minimal shoes would be better. The only problem I have with my treadmill is that I have to be aware of my form and adjustments that I need to make, because my treadmill is bouncy. Still, I would rather run on a treadmill than not run at all.

As a mom, do you ever run with a running stroller? Is it difficult to see obstacles or pebbles in your path?

Angie: I do. It's a really great workout – to put a kid in there, and push him around.

I have to be careful, so I don't go as fast, but you don't have to run directly behind the stroller. You can run next to it and still steer it so you can see where you're going. Run next to it and back off a little, and you can steer it with one hand if you have it balanced right.

Do you have any suggestions for barefoot beginners?

Angie: When I first started barefoot running, the hardest part was getting out the door – just getting going. I would come up with all kinds of excuses: I have laundry to do, I have to prepare this meal, things to do on the computer. All these excuses, but every single time I've gone, I was glad I did.

I really enjoy running. It's just so good for me on so many levels. It's an incredible stress reliever as a parent. It gives me something that's my own. In turn, it helps my family, and we are all better because of it. It's something I take pride in and I work at.

It was really incredible to give birth and nurse my sons— it was such a natural thing to do. I didn't have to learn any of it. Of course, I did *read* about it, just as I read about barefoot running. When it comes down to it, your body is designed to do all these things. And if you just have faith that your body will do it, your body will find its way. But it can be hard to let go and trust that your body knows what it's doing.

Final thoughts?

Angie: If you are not having fun, what is the point? When I was running in shoes, I wanted to like running – the idea of being outside, the motions. I *wanted* to like it, but I didn't.

Now, I have these friends who go through marathon training. And they push so hard and stick to this rigid schedule. I would say at least three-quarters of them, if not more, all shod runners, they get injured within their training cycle. And the bloggers, you know, they blog about hating to run, and so many of them don't like it.

I honestly cannot think of a run that I didn't enjoy. If anything, I might have been tired or not gotten much sleep, but I always felt better when I got there. I think it has to do with my feet and the feedback I get from them. I am so much more in tune with my surroundings, and it makes me happier. For that reason alone, it's more fun.

Kids ask me, "Why are you running barefoot?"

Ninety-nine percent of the time, I say, "It's more fun to run without shoes." Then you can see the lights go on. Kids are easy to get in touch with once you tell them it's more fun.

Is This Even Legal?

Is this even legal? Should I expect to run into "no shoes, no service" problems?

Running barefoot outdoors is perfectly legal. As for indoors, private establishments can make their own rules, and unfortunately many gyms do disallow bare feet, often based on a mistaken understanding of health codes.

If you are ever barred from a store or gym for not wearing shoes, you may want to remind them, as nicely as possible, that they are losing the dollars you would have spent there.

What about in road races?

In the U.S., I've never heard of an open (non-scholastic) road race that required shoes.

During a race, we push our bodies to the limit while running on unfamiliar terrain. Some surfaces are more barefoot friendly than others, so it pays to check out the race course beforehand. That's always good race strategy – not just when running barefoot.

When I run a race without shoes and shoelaces, how will I attach my timing chip?

Triathletes wear their tags on a Velcro strap, available for a few dollars at many sporting goods stores. These work well.

The tag must be close to the ground. Do not hold it in your hand or put it in your skort pocket.

My kid's coach requires him to wear shoes.

Yes, things are different at the scholastic and inter-collegiate level. Many coaches, believing they are protecting their charges, require shoes, as do some athletic conferences.

Many scholastic and collegiate runners incur serious and long-lasting injuries due to the pressures of shod competitive running. Perhaps better education will help to change these outmoded and harmful attitudes.

What about triathlons?

In the Netherlands, shoes are apparently required in the running leg of a triathlon. Fortunately, this type of regulation is rare. Check with the race organizer.

This feels like a New Age fad. I'm not sure I trust it. Does the Bible mention barefoot running?

Well, not "running" per se. However, let's take a look at Exodus 3:4-5:

> When the Lord saw that he had gone over to look, God called to him from within the bush, "Moses! Moses!" And Moses said, "Here I am."

> "Do not come any closer," God said. "Take off your sandals, for the place where you are standing is holy ground."

Seems pretty clear to me. The earth is holy ground. Why step on it with your shoes? Why are all these other people telling you to wear shoes?

Summary: Yes it is legal.

What About Normal Running Injuries?

What about normal running injuries – you know, the painful non-fatal injuries that we all suffer. How does barefoot running affect those?

You're leading me to my main point. Most of the injuries that runners accept as a "normal" and unavoidable part of the running experience, are not unavoidable at all. You suffer them because you wear shoes, not because you run.

Blistered and bloody toes?

Only from banging up against the front of your running shoes. You should see the blood blisters on the toes of some of my shod marathon-running friends!

Doesn't happen to barefoot runners.

Blackened and broken toenails?

Nope. That also only happens because of toes banging against shoes.

One friend lost six toenails after running the recent Chicago Marathon. But to her and to many other shod runners, that seems completely normal.

Why is losing toenails considered normal? And if that much pain and unpleasantness is acceptable, why such fear of a splinter every few months?

Corns and bunions?

Not if you're barefoot. Bunions (hallux valgus) and corns are shoe-induced. I know from past experience that they are unattractive, very painful, and expensive to remove. Why would you choose to have them? [PAPER11]

Sprained ankles?

This is a common but serious injury that has put two of my running friends on crutches for months at a time. It can be much worse than the very unlikely stepping-on-a-nail injury, or even than a foot stress fracture.

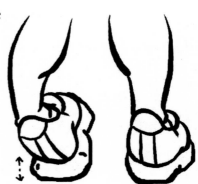

By restricting the natural movement of your feet and ankles, shoes increase the likelihood of ankle injuries. [PAPER6]

When you twist your ankle by tripping over the side of your shoe, the rotational force on your ankle is a product of your weight and the height of the sole of your shoe. But when you're barefoot, there's no sole to "fall off of." Therefore, no sprained ankle.

Untied shoelaces mid-race?

An annoyance, rather than an injury, this is a surprisingly common problem for shod runners. And it never happens when you're barefoot.

What are the most frequent shod-running injuries?

In addition to the foot and ankle injuries listed above, shod runners frequently suffer from:

- ► Shin splints.
- ► Runner's knee.
- ► Plantar fasciitis.
- ► Iliotiobial Band Syndrome (ITBS).
- ► Achilles tendonitis.

During my shod running career, I endured all of these injuries, sometimes sidelined for more than a year at a time.

Most active runners suffer an injury every year. And that includes only those who stay healthy enough to stick with running. A large number of one-time runners drop out of the sport due to chronic injury.

I meet injured twenty- and thirty-something runners, including former competitive athletes, who've been told that they've "destroyed" their knee joints, and will never be able to run again.

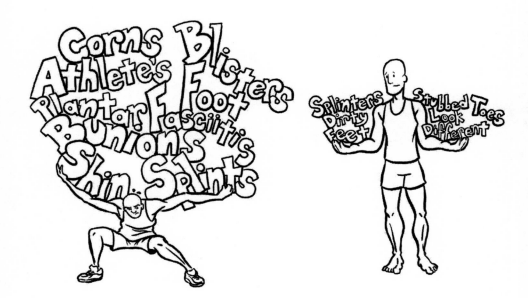

That just can't be natural. It must be the result of doing something very wrong. And that "something wrong" is running with the equivalent of blindfolds on your feet, deadening yourself to sensation, and allowing yourself to abuse your body far beyond its natural limits.

Barefoot running is about getting back in touch with your body and your surroundings, so that you can use, not abuse, your physical gifts over a long and healthy life.

Summary: Many commonly accepted "running injuries" are primarily "shoe wearer's injuries."

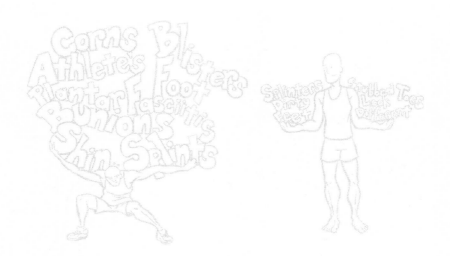

Interview:

Barefoot TJ: "Join The Barefoot Runners Society And Quit The Running Injured Club"

And you are …?

Tamara Gerken. My friends call me Barefoot TJ. I'm 44, married with two young boys, and I live in the metro Atlanta area.

I've been running for over six years, and the last two have been barefoot. I first began running for fitness, and didn't really care for it, but after I shed the shoes, I absolutely fell in love with running … barefoot.

What attracted you to barefoot running?

Barefoot TJ: I have Morton's neuroma, two in each foot. It is extremely painful. I developed this condition as a direct result of the shoes I wore in the past, and I'm unable to run in shoes anymore.

I can't run in shoes. Barefoot, I can run 17 miles.

What were your concerns about bare-footing?

Barefoot TJ: I had none. Knowing how much pain I was going through with running shoes, I figured running barefoot couldn't be any worse. In fact, it's been so much better.

How was the transition?

Barefoot TJ: I didn't have any trouble transitioning. It would have been quicker if I had resolved to leave the shoes entirely behind after that first barefoot run, but as so many of us do, I was convinced that running shoes were a requirement for running.

What surprised you – good or bad?

Barefoot TJ: I enjoyed the sense of freedom that came from shedding the weight of the shoes. Running is no longer a chore. It's something that I want to do – that I'm eager to do. And I don't have to worry about whether my clothes match my shoes.

Tips for beginners?

Barefoot TJ: Don't be so concerned about how others are running and what their form looks like, but instead concentrate on your own form, a form that will most likely be unique to you. The way to do this is to actually listen to your body and feel the ground through your feet. The quickest way and safest way to transition to barefoot running is to ditch the shoes cold turkey and make the necessary sacrifices to your speed and distance upfront. Transitioning slowly while running part-time in shoes will only take you that much longer.

Also, start by walking around barefoot every day. Go everywhere you can barefoot, and stay barefoot as much as possible. After a run, look at the bottom of your feet closely. Look for signs of blisters. If you are developing blisters on the balls of your feet, then you are pushing off. Instead, lift your feet. If you are developing blisters on your heels, then you are heel striking. Instead, lean over your center of gravity, and bend your knees more. The wear patterns on your feet will not only tell you where you've been, they will also tell you how you got there.

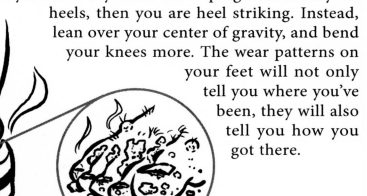

Don't your feet get dirty?

Barefoot TJ: My feet are a lot cleaner now than when I used to shove them in a pair of smelly, sweaty shoes. At least with bare feet, your sweat evaporates. In shoes, the sweat just accumulates and grows pools of bacteria.

What about arch support?

Barefoot TJ: I used to have flat feet, and I "overpronated." Now I have a nice arch. Since I've built up my arch muscles, my feet have lifted, and I no longer pronate as much as I used to. My feet also seem to have widened in the forefoot.

Doesn't it hurt?

Barefoot TJ: Not really. Once you've done it awhile, it's like anything else: it gets easier. In fact, I have never experienced a barefoot running-related injury. I just listened to my body, and allowed my feet to tell me how far and how fast to go.

What surfaces do you run on?

Barefoot TJ: Asphalt mostly, but I love trail running when I can. When I run trails, I naturally slow down, but I get to really enjoy the different textures and sensations I receive from the ground.

What about the cold?

Barefoot TJ: You can train yourself to tolerate the cold. I have learned my limitations in the cold, and what I have found is that I can run down to 27 degrees Fahrenheit when it is dry, and any temps over 40 degrees when it is wet. You can also try to save your runs for the warmest part of the day.

Does it feel icky?

Barefoot TJ: Quite the opposite. It "feels," and there's nothing better than to feel alive.

How has your family reacted?

Barefoot TJ: They have grown very supportive. I even think my husband is proud of his oddball wife's barefoot running.

Do you think this is a fad?

Barefoot TJ: I believe this is more of a movement than a fad. People are just starting to recognize that the traditional running shoes we've been wearing for the past 30-plus years are unnecessary and possibly the cause of many injuries. People are tired of running in pain. They are now learning there are alternatives.

I do believe, however, that the number of people running barefoot will never equal the number of people running shod. I fully expect the minimalist footwear-running movement to take off. It's important to note, though, that if it weren't for the barefoot running movement, there would never have been a minimalist footwear-running movement.

I encourage runners to join the Barefoot Runners Society (BarefootRunners.org) and quit the running injured club!

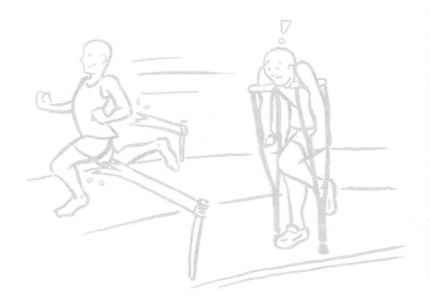

How Do I Get Started?

How do I get started?

It's very easy. Find a clean, hard surface – the shoulder or bike lane of a road, or a sidewalk. Take off your shoes and run. The road and your feet are all you need.

Also, start small. As long as you listen to your body, the sensitivity of your skin will limit how far you can run. Your skin will gradually become less sensitive, allowing you to run farther. This gradual increase in weekly mileage will allow the muscles, tendons and ligaments of your feet the time they need to adapt to an unfamiliar activity.

Part of barefoot running is watching the road ahead, and watching where you put your feet. Barefoot running is mindful running – keen awareness of your surroundings and of the experience. That means looking and listening. No music.

No music?

No music – especially not in the initial learning period. Pay attention to the running path and the feedback from your feet.

How do I prepare? Do I need to strengthen my feet?

Your feet do not need any special preparation. Over millions of years, they have evolved to support your body as you walk or run. Your feet cause problems only when you get in their way – by cramming them into rigid shoes that restrict their freedom of movement and impose an un-naturally hot and humid environment.

What's the best way to transition – how long does it take?

This depends on how much you run. If you are running up to 20 miles a week, you may want to allow three to four months to regain your mileage. If you are running 50 to 70 miles a week, which is the most I've ever run, allow at least six months. During this period, do not do any fast/track running. You may be itching to show off your bare toes to the running community, but it's best not to rush it. Also keep in mind that people adapt at different rates.

For the competitive runners among you, six months means missing an entire season. Then again, if you are chronically injured, you wouldn't be racing very much anyway.

To summarize, your basic transition plan is this: take off your shoes and do it! The beauty of barefoot running is that it is self-governing. The initial tenderness of your skin limits how far you go and thereby reduces the risk of hurting yourself by doing too much, too soon. Your skin toughens up as your feet strengthen. Listen to your body as you increase mileage, and in six months or so, you'll be back to your previous running program and more.

Can anybody start barefoot running right away, or are there cases where it's better to slowly move from shod running to barefoot running?

When developing any new habit, it's best to practice only that habit, and not continue to reinforce the old, bad ways. I recommend that you start running barefoot and *only* barefoot.

Yes, this will mean sharply reducing your total mileage for a few months. The payoff is a long and healthy lifetime of running.

What should I watch out for?

Walking around in typical shoes with elevated heels has probably shortened your calf muscles and thickened and stiffened your Achilles tendons. [PAPER17] This is reversible, but the transition to no heels should be made very gently. Pain in the Achilles region is a warning to take it easy.

Will I need to change my training routine?

Most recreational runners can train just as hard barefoot as they did shod. Many find, as I did, that we can train much harder, since our chronic injuries have melted away.

The lessons here are aimed at adult fitness runners, rather than youthful sprinters.

I have a marathon next month and have been training in shoes. Should I change now?

No. Though I don't encourage running a marathon in built-up shoes, wait until after the big race before changing anything about your equipment.

I've never run. Can I do this?

Yes, barefoot running is available to everyone. Lucky you to be spared the expense and pain of running in shoes! Check with your physician before starting a program of rigorous exercise.

A full intro-to-running program is beyond the scope of this book. Finding a running community is a great way to start. Perhaps you have neighbors or friends who already run; perhaps your town has a running club. When I resumed running after a multi-year layoff (because of IT Band Syndrome), it was with a great organization called Team in Training, which I highly recommend.

What's the farthest I should run barefoot?

As far as you want. Running is great for your health, whether you run three or four times a week, or train for a marathon (26.2 miles). Just listen to your body.

The limiting factor is not your shoes or lack thereof, but your desire to keep running when you could be home, feet up, watching reruns of *Star Trek*.

Summary: Start out slow. Listen to your body.

Interview:

John Stieber:
"To Be 60 And Feel Like A Kid Again Is Pretty Good"

And you are ...?

John Stieber. I'm 60 years old, and I live in Menlo Park, California.

Will you take us through your running history?

John: I ran cross country in high school, and then I started running again in 2002. I took a Chi Running course in 2004, and ran a marathon in the summer. My time wasn't spectacular, but I enjoyed it.

What I found is that shoes were always a problem for me.

I tried different brands, different sizes, and I would have blisters. I'd get pain across the bottom of my feet, and my left Achilles tendon would start to hurt pretty regularly. I would listen to people saying, "You should get more shoes, more stability, lifts in your shoes." I even bought a pair of running orthotics, and I finally found I could wear Brooks shoes. They were pretty comfortable – there is just something about the wider toe box in Brooks shoes. But even though I was running without blisters in the forefoot [in Brooks], I had pain in my Achilles tendon – from top to bottom.

How are your feet? Healthy?

John: I'm very flat footed – always have been. I started off in these very heavy motion-control shoes. They were very heavy and clunky, and I didn't enjoy running in them.

So then I went to a workshop by Danny Dreyer. He's the guy who came up with Chi Running. He was recommending minimalist running shoes, and suggested a model of Adidas shoe from the 1970s. But I started to get blisters again. I ran three more marathons – in '06, '07 and one in '08. I was going to run one in '09, but I broke my kneecap while backpacking. It hurt for a while, and it's hard getting out of the backcountry, believe me. Fortunately, it was a nice clean break, and it healed without surgery, but it really threw everything off.

Back when I was looking for minimalist shoes, I tried the Nike Free. I went through a few pairs, but they completely fell apart. I would take them back, get my money back, and buy a new pair, but it's just the way they were made. A friend was wearing Nike Frees, and they exacerbated a number of injuries for her – ankles, heels and knees.

Then in the summer of '09, I read *Born to Run*, and immediately got a visceral, "Ah hah! I can run without shoes!"

I literally did what the guy in this book did. I went out one day, and ran about half a mile, at most. I felt playful – like a child.

How has it been since then?

John: Rediscovering running in my early fifties, and finding the freedom to run without shoes, has just been great. I went to a workshop at Zombie Runner [local running store] on barefoot running, and Barefoot Ted and Chris McDougall came. They offered reassurance that this is something you can do comfortably and safely. Not only is it not bad for you, it's actually good for you.

Many people wonder whether they are too old to start barefoot running. Any thoughts on that?

John: I'm 60 years old, and it has rejuvenated me. I like to run correctly, have fun, and not hurt myself.

I eased into it. Technique is very important, but I think it's true that running barefoot almost makes you run properly.

Older people who are very active, who have had surgeries - their knees aren't what they used to be. But I don't see how this will hurt anything. As [Pose Method teacher] Lee Saxby said, if the mechanics are right, almost anyone should be able to run barefoot.

To sustain anything, there has to be some inherent joy. You should look forward to the experience, and that only happens if you're doing it correctly – if you're not injuring yourself, if you're getting more energy from it.

For people who are burned out – not just physically but mentally – it's like resetting everything. It's like starting over. To be 60 and feel like a kid again is pretty good.

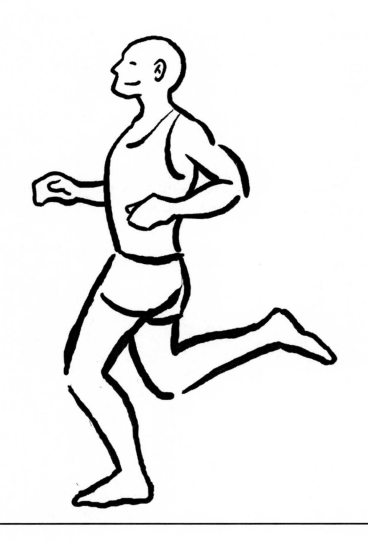

Remember: Bend Your Knees

Transitioning To Barefoot:
A Plan

DAY 0: Preparing To Run

- ▸ Take a few pictures of your feet, or have someone else take pictures. Note the lighting so that you can reproduce it.
- ▸ Also take pictures of your wet footprint.
- ▸ How do your feet look and feel to you? Do they feel strong? Do they smell? Do you feel they are attractive or unattractive? Is the skin smooth or rough? Are the soles callused? Do you have corns or bunions? How are the toenails? Are you proud or ashamed to display your feet? Do you wish they looked different? How?

Write down your observations and thoughts.

Day 0: Being Barefoot

- ► If you wear shoes in the house, get in the habit of being barefoot. Once this feels comfortable, take a walk around the block barefoot, or for a few blocks. Don't listen to music. Listen to your body.
- ► Get in the habit of leaving socks by the door, so you don't track dirt into your home.
- ► When you must wear shoes, choose footwear without raised heels and rigid soles.

Day 1: The First Run

- ► Start indoors. Stand behind a chair, holding on to the back, and very gently run in place. Think about raising your feet using your hamstrings (back of your thighs), and do *not* push off your feet.
- ► Think about standing tall. One benefit of running behind a chair is that it reduces the tendency to lean forward.
- ► Think about "letting" your knees move forward as you lift your feet.
- ► Do this movement behind the chair for a few minutes. Really feel it. Then turn around, make your way to the door, step outside, and continue.

Congratulations! You are officially a barefoot runner. Yes, it really is that natural, that easy.

Write down your experience.

_____

_____

_____

_____

_____

_____

_____

_____

Week 1 - 3: Exploration

▸ Run no more than one to two miles barefoot, three times. Take it very easy. Relax your whole body. Stand tall. Bend your knees. Lift your feet (do not push off). How does it feel?

▸ Observe the road surface with your eyes and with your feet. What do you notice that you didn't see before? (I had never noticed that sidewalks were squares of concrete – often broken!)

▸ You will stub your toe. You will step on pebbles and acorns. You can curse me – it's okay. How long does the pain last?

▸ You may feel hot spots (pre-blisters) on the soles of your feet. Either you are running on a very hot summer road (stick to the white lines), or more likely, you are pushing off with your feet. Resist the urge to push. Lift your feet. Consider ending today's run.

▸ If your Achilles tendon and calf muscles feel un-comfortably tight, be very conscious of maintaining an upright position and *not* leaning forward. Don't forget to do the foam roller exercises described in the Stretching chapter.

▸ Before going to sleep, pamper your feet with a hot Epsom salts soak or a massage.

Week 4 - 5: Familiarisation

▸ Run two to three miles barefoot, three times. Take it easy. How does it feel?

▸ Lift your feet. Bend your knees. Don't push off.

▸ If the soles of your feet hurt, or especially if you feel pain on the top of your feet, call it quits for the day.

Weeks 6+: Ingraining Good Form

- ► If you wish, increase your mileage gradually.
- ► Lift your feet. Bend your knees. Don't push off.

Months 2 - 6: Solidifying The Foundation

- ► Do not race, even if you are tempted or your friends encourage you. Stick to easy running on clean, clear roads and sidewalks. Do not set yourself any goal other than to enjoy this new movement form. Savor the ground under your feet.
- ► What comments do you receive from passersby? How do you react to them? Do you feel special?
- ► How does it feel to run on a hot or cold or wet or rough surface?
- ► Are you remembering to lift your feet and bend your knees?

At The 6 Month Point

- ► Redo the Day 0 exercise – photos and all. How have your feet changed? Does your footprint look different? What about the skin on the soles of your feet?

_____
_____
_____
_____
_____
_____
_____
_____
_____
_____
_____
_____
_____

Months 7 - 12

- ▶ The novelty should have worn off. Perhaps you are no longer even conscious of being "different" from other runners. By now you have grown accustomed to running without nagging injuries and pain.
- ▶ Reread the book. Do you relate to the experience of the other runners? Are you practicing good form? Are you following the stretching and strengthening recommendations?
- ▶ Remember Zola Budd and Abebe Bikila. Remember the hundreds of thousands of years that your ancestors ran barefoot.

Just run.

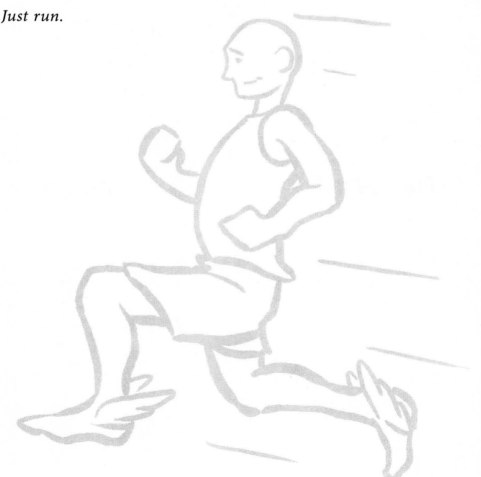

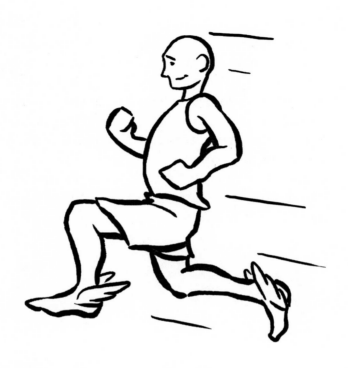

Remember: Take Quick Light Steps

Do I Run On My Toes Or On My Heels?

Do I run on my toes or on my heels?

Neither. Good form is what your body discovers for itself when your feet feel the ground. I can promise that you won't run barefoot on your heels for more than two steps!

So I run on my toes?

No. Actually, this is a common question, and important to clarify. *Do not force yourself to run up on the front of your feet.* I saw someone doing this the other day, in shoes. It looked awkward, painful, and very unnatural. It will lead to injury.

So which is it?!

If you saw me running, you'd think I was running flat-footed. But don't try to imitate me or any other runner. Run barefoot on hard ground, bend your knees, and don't push off. Your natural footfall is best.

Just relax as you run. Don't force yourself into any particular form.

When you run relaxed, you will most likely land on your mid-foot or with slightly more pressure on the front half of your foot than on the back. But, and I can't stress this enough, don't "try" to do that! Just let it happen.

Is it okay for my heels to touch the ground?

If your heels naturally touch the ground during your stride, that is absolutely fine. In fact, unless you are sprinting, it is very likely.

I've been running for years. Why should I change my natural form?

You may be reading this book because your current running form has led to injuries, and you'd like to be healthy again.

If you've been running in cushioned shoes with a thick heel counter, your form is nothing like "natural." Those high heels restrict and distort your body's natural movement patterns.

The good news is that you can rediscover natural form for yourself, by removing what gets in the way – the shoes.

To what extent will going barefoot change the way I run?

Running shoeless on a hard surface encourages you to run with good form – the way your body was designed to move.

How much of a change will it be? It depends on how you run today. Modern "stability" shoes with built-up heels force a heel strike landing. Barefoot, your weight will land forward of the heel.

To see how shoes force a natural forefoot striker to land on her heel, watch [VIDEO2]:

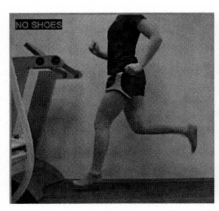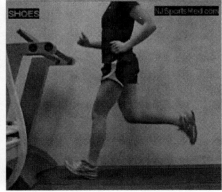

How can I find perfect running form?

Perfection is hard to achieve. Your natural barefoot running stride, even if imperfect, should allow you a lifetime of running, free of serious injury. [VIDEO2]

Remember to bend your knees, lift your feet (don't push off), and stand tall (don't lean forward).

How will I know when I'm doing it right?

When you get it right, good form feels like running downhill. On a good day, I have this downhill sensation through my entire six-mile neighborhood loop, as if running in a giant Escher painting. It's a wonderful feeling.

On a more basic level, doing it right means running injury-free for the long term. If you are already achieving the mileage and pace that you want, injury free, I won't suggest that you change anything.

I like a powerful stride. How can I achieve that?

This is a misunderstanding of running form. The sense of power you get from pounding the ground can be exhilarating in a sprint, but will wear out your body in the long run – as you're already discovering.

Another thing: vertical energy is wasted energy, and it also leads to unnecessary pounding on your joints. Some runners wear a pendant against their chest while running. If the pendant doesn't move, their form is smooth. If it bounces, they are bouncing too much.

Okay, I get it. Listen to my body, run lightly without impact. Can you enumerate all the elements of good running form?

1. Consciously relax your body, including the shoulders, hands and feet.

2. Stand tall. Do not slouch or collapse.

3. Bend your knees.

4. Do not push off with your feet. Do not "toe off."

5. Think of pulling your feet up using the hamstring (back of legs) muscles, rather than driving forward with your knees.

6. Minimize ground contact time. Think about pulling up even as your feet are just touching down.

7. Keep your head in a neutral position, neither looking down at your feet nor craning up with a tense neck.

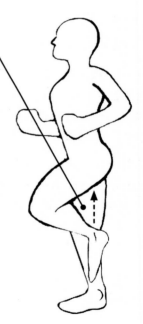

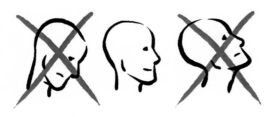

8. Think of taking quick, light steps – flowing and floating, rather than powerful or pounding. Your feet should make little or no sound as they contact the ground.

9. Resist the temptation to lean forward. In particular, do not lean forward at the hips.

10. You have achieved the Holy Grail of good running form when your foot lands under you, not in front of you. This is difficult in practice, but you can get close – think of pushing forward with your hips (without arching your back) as you run.

You recommend standing tall. How can I move forward if I don't lean forward?

Some coaches do advise leaning forward from the ankles, but in my experience, if you can feel the lean, it's already too much.

Over-leaning from the ankle can cause strain on the Achilles tendon and calf muscles.

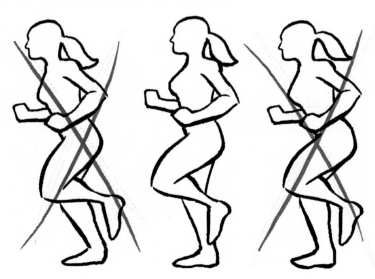

Leaning from the hips throws off your form entirely, and is a major error.

In short, over-leaning causes many more problems than "not leaning enough" – if there is such a thing. Focus on standing tall and relaxed, neither straining nor collapsing.

Why should I land with my feet under me? I see so many pictures of runners landing with a straight knee and one foot far ahead of them.

That is called "overstriding," and you see the most extreme examples in advertising – not among runners who stay healthy for very long.

Think about what happens when you over-stride. When you slam your feet into the ground, you are braking your body with each step. In addition to the shock waves pulsing through your legs, does constant braking sound efficient?

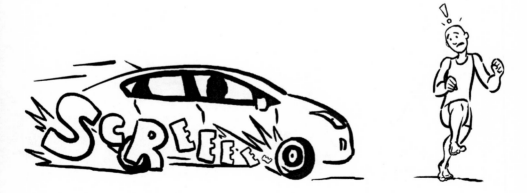

The Toyota Prius generates energy through regenerative braking. You don't.

We're all different. Why should we all run the same way?

Every tennis coach teaches students to use body mass to power a serve. No tennis coach in the world teaches students to power through a serve with the biceps.

Every piano teacher instructs pupils to keep their hands and arms relaxed. No piano teacher in the world tells students to keep their fingers stiff and rigid, or to wear thick rubber gloves "for protection" from the keys.

So yes, the shapes of our bodies may differ, but a few principles are common to good (and bad) movement.

Your body will find good form when you run barefoot on a hard surface, standing tall yet relaxed, staying conscious of bending your knees, and lifting (not pushing) your feet. Your mission is to let it happen without getting in the way.

And yes, we are different, and your exact cadence, stride length and foot-impact point will vary according to your body and your pace.

I read that most runners heel strike.

It certainly is possible that most runners heel strike when wearing running shoes with built-up heels. The thick heel sticks out and more or less forces a heel-first landing. That doesn't make it right. Thick rubber heels muffle the impact, but they don't prevent the shock from moving up your shins, knees and back. [VIDEO4]

What are the benefits of forefoot versus mid-foot strike?

Those are just labels. Try to run with good form, and observe (don't try to change) how your feet contact the ground. On most days it will feel like a mid-foot strike, but it will vary according to your speed on any given day.

What do you think about Chi Running, Evolution Running, and the Pose Method?

I have studied most of the well-known running techniques, in many cases taking instruction directly from the founders. It was a mixed bag. The Pose Method stands out for its deep insights, but at the end of the day, I found I benefited most from just taking off my shoes and running. It doesn't require lots of theory and rules and book learning.

One prolific running author (a shrill opponent of barefoot running) recommends actively driving your foot into the ground – the harder, the better. I won't even bother with the science on this one. Take it from me: if you want a long and healthy life, don't slam your feet into the ground. While you're at it, stay away from punching light poles with your fist or breaking concrete blocks with your forehead.

My running coach and many books tell me that running form can't be taught or changed. Your natural form is what it is.

In a way, I agree. If you didn't interfere with your body's natural movement patterns by loading up your feet with a block of hard rubber that lifts your heels an inch off the ground, and artificially cants your hips forward, you wouldn't need to be taught form. You would just run, and you'd be fine. [ARTICLE1]

I've heard that I should maintain a cadence of at least 180 steps per minute. Is that true? Should I run with a metronome?

Yes and no. It is true that a cadence below 180 (90 steps per foot per minute) indicates that your form may need tweaking. However, the way to improve your form is to focus directly on *form* – not on cadence. You do not want to force your cadence higher by pushing hard. That will get you nowhere, except (possibly) injured.

If you follow my guidance, you shouldn't have to worry about cadence. I suggest you forget the metronome, because it will get you thinking and counting, distracting you from feeling the fluid movement of your body.

Mathematically speaking, form is the independent variable, and cadence is the dependent variable.

What is bad running form?

I'd rather you think about good form, so bend your knees, maintain upright posture, and pull your feet up, rather than pushing off.

Just so you can learn from the mistakes of others, typical injury-provoking form errors include:

- Landing with your feet far in front of your body – on your heels, with your knees locked. This is the classic running-shoe advertising pose, and it's a killer.

- Taking big, slow, heavy steps, feeling the pounding in your back and neck. I used to run like this. I knew something was wrong, but I didn't know what, or how to change. Cushioned running shoes really encourage this style.

- Pushing off with your feet. Easy mistake to make, and fortunately easy to fix.

- Pawback. Related to the push off - trying to pull the ground back behind you on each step. Just say no.

- Driving forward or upward with your knees. No, no, no.

- Leaning forward from the hips, sometimes called a K-bend. This is an easy mistake to make, particularly if you have been told to lean forward.

- ▸ "Sitting in a bucket," with your butt sticking out behind you – often the consequence of a K-bend.

- ▸ Slapping the ground with your feet. Loud sound is a dead giveaway of poor form. Sound means that your feet are hitting the ground hard, and the resulting impact force will penetrate up to hurt your shins and knees.

Running down hills always gives me shin splints. Will it be worse without the cushioning?

Running downhill doesn't require cushioning, but it does require good technique and careful practice.

The trick (as before) is to bend your knees, and to take very short, quick steps, with higher cadence than on level ground, almost flowing downhill. You don't want to fight gravity, nor do you want to streak downhill with huge, bounding strides.

Try to land with your feet under you, rather than out in front of you. Do not lean back and brake with each step. Braking may feel superficially safer, but it creates more impact, leading to injury.

When I have a wide path, sometimes I will zigzag down a hill rather than run straight down. Don't do this on a path shared with bicyclists or faster runners.

Years ago, while still running shod, I took an hour of downhill running lessons with a well-known running coach, and ended up with shin splints a week before a big race. Practice a little at a time.

What about running uphill?

Take shorter, quicker steps when running uphill – just like changing into a lower gear on a bicycle.

Very consciously think of pulling your feet up with every step, and avoid the temptation to push. I literally think of "pulling myself up the hill." It is a great opportunity to practice technique.

On uphills as on downhills, be conscious of relaxing your body, and not tensing with the effort. It may help to consciously relax your face.

What's the mechanical difference between running barefoot and in minimal shoes?

Feedback. The sensation that your foot receives from each step allows your body to continually adapt and adjust.

Even the most minimal shoe reduces feedback to your feet. Once you've learned and internalized good form, a minimal shoe (the type worn by most elite runners) won't stop you from running properly. However, while you're still learning to run, shoes get in the way.

What about my breathing?

Good question. Keep your mouth closed, and breathe exclusively through a device specifically designed for breathing – your nose.

In the early stages of barefoot running, nasal breathing will help you slow to a safe pace. Keeping your mouth closed may also help your neck position. An open jaw throws off the balance of the head.

At first, this definitely feels unnatural, but I encourage you to persevere. I've used my nose for breathing on many 20-mile runs. I find that it helps regulate my pace, so I don't huff and puff (hyperventilate) and wear myself out early.

Nasal breathing is also taught in yoga, and was recommended by Ukrainian physician Konstantin Buteyko to cure asthma – his teachings have quite a following.

What about my head and neck?

Keep your neck in a neutral position, neither bent back nor craned forward like an ostrich.

You need to see yourself from the side, which is tough to do in a mirror. It may help to watch yourself on video, or have a friend spot you.

Which muscles do I use when I run?

I encourage you to focus on maintaining fluid movement, rather than think about specific muscles.

Do think of lifting your feet up, rather than driving upward with your knees or pushing off with your feet.

Summary: Relax. Bend your knees. Lift your feet.

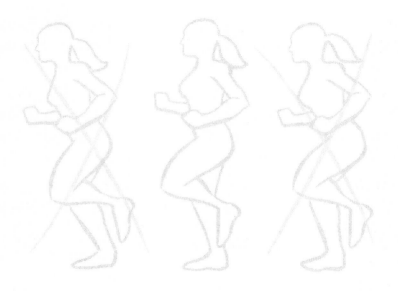

Is This A Guy Thing?

Is this a guy thing? Women didn't necessarily evolve to run after wild animals. We were home, taking care of the kids, while the men hunted.

The studies on barefoot running were conducted on women and men, and the results apply equally.

Women can and do enjoy the benefits of barefoot running, from better overall health to prettier toes. Read my interviews with Cassie, Angie, TJ and Heather.

Is there a difference in impact forces between men versus women?

Published research shows similar data for women and men regarding the impact forces experienced during shod and unshod running.

Can pregnant women run barefoot?

Yes, assuming they have the green light from their doctors. Judge for yourself whether to engage in a new physical activity during pregnancy. It's a personal choice.

As women's bodies change during pregnancy, and as their center of gravity moves, keeping good form becomes more important than ever.

One female contributor to the *Runner's World* barefoot forum suggested that pregnancy could be a great time to begin barefoot walking. The shape of the feet change, and as she put it, "There's a reason for the phrase 'barefoot and pregnant.'"

Since my feet spread during pregnancy (due to relaxation of the tendons), is it okay to start barefoot running right after giving birth, or should I wait until I'm done breastfeeding (when most of the hormones that cause relaxation are gone)?

As above, run if you are comfortable doing so. Perhaps start by walking barefoot. If you feel okay and have your doctor's okay, it is okay to run barefoot.

One barefoot runner wrote to me that the loosening of her tendons required her to slow way down during pregnancy. On the plus side, many women achieve their best performances after childbirth.

What about running behind a running stroller?

For men and women alike, it's important to see where your feet are landing. So, as you push that stroller, be sure to scan the ground ahead of it.

In her interview, Angie B suggests running slightly to one side of the stroller, to control it while also maintaining a view ahead.

Is running barefoot feminine?

Consider the other extreme: high heels. Some think that heels empower women, and others that they oppress.

Is living in pain feminine, or is pain-free good health feminine? Only you can decide for yourself.

Summary: Running barefoot benefits women and men alike.

Interview:

Heather Wiatrowski:
"... First Summer Since I've Been A Runner That I've Been Able To Wear Sandals"

And you are ...?

Heather Wiatrowski. I am a professor in the biology department at Clark University in Worcester, Massachusetts.

I hear you're a barefoot runner. How did you arrive at this?

Heather: By October 2009, I was really frustrated with my running shoes. They had been irritating my Achilles region, and I couldn't go four miles before I ended up bloody. The model of shoe I'd been wearing for six years wasn't working for me anymore. I'd been going through new pairs of shoes, trying new models, and nothing felt right. After running about six miles in my last pair of shoes, which felt okay in the store, everything hurt – my ankles, shins, knees, hips, back, and even my shoulders and my head.

Wow.

Heather: I was at a low point when I saw an article about Christopher McDougall and *Born to Run* in *The New York Times*. Since I was so frustrated with my shoes, I figured I'd just try barefooting. So, I ran around my block barefoot. My block is only a quarter of a mile long, and I was expecting it to be really uncomfortable and painful, but it wasn't. It turned out to be fine. So, I ran around the block again, and it was fine, and I ran around the block a third time, and it was still fine, and onwards and upwards from there.

When you say barefoot, do you mean in minimalist shoes?

Heather: Oh no. I read the article on Christopher McDougall at 4:00 in the afternoon (at work), and by 5:30 in the evening, I was running outside. I didn't buy any shoes. I didn't put anything on my feet. I just got my running clothes on, and I just skipped the part ankles down.

That's pretty gutsy. For me, even after doing some reading, there was a lot of hesitation.

Heather: Well, it was just around the block, so I figured if it was terrible, I'd come right back. It's not like I had to run five miles before I could stop.

How has it gone since that first day?

Heather: It took a little over six weeks to get the hang of it. I had a couple of blisters starting out, behind my second toe, but those went away after about two months. I haven't had a problem with that since. After about three months, my mileage was increasing, and I was running faster. I felt great, and I was running a whole lot more than I had before I started running barefoot.

Don't your feet get dirty?

Heather: Not nearly as dirty as you'd think - I've never left tracks in the house. If it's recently rained, sometimes they come back a little muddy, but it's nothing that can't be dealt with pretty quickly – like by rubbing them on the mat in the breezeway.

How does your family feel about this?

Heather: It's funny. My kids didn't know. They're five and seven, and they hadn't noticed that I was running barefoot. They were both informed by their teachers, who had seen me running barefoot. They asked the kids, "Is that your mom, the lady who runs barefoot?" And they came home, and asked me, "Mom do you run barefoot?" Now they think it's kind of cool.

And your husband?

Heather: We were betting on whether my feet would turn into hobbit feet. You have to understand that they looked really bad before I started barefoot running because my Achilles region was all torn up from the previous shoes. I'd lost a couple of toenails – standard things that happen to runners. I had classic runners' feet, and they didn't look good at all, but after I started barefoot running, I didn't have that irritation from the shoes.

Now, my feet look really, really good. This past summer was the first summer since I've been a runner that I've been able to wear sandals. My toenails all looked perfect.

So your feet no longer bleed from the shoes, your body no longer hurts all over, your toenails look great. What else do you like about barefoot running?

Heather: It's nice not to have to carry shoes with me to work if I'm going to run at lunch. Shoes are heavy, and when I would travel, I'd always wonder whether to carry them on the airplane. I'd think, "Can I fit the running shoes?" Now, I don't have to worry about that. I put my running gear in a tiny bag. That was another unexpected benefit.

Any last words of advice? How have your interactions been with other runners?

Heather: Mostly, it's been pretty positive. Occasionally, I run into older men who behave in a very paternalistic way toward me. They warn me that I'm going to hurt myself, and that can get a little frustrating, so I usually just run away. It *is* a race – after all. That's the nice thing about a race. You can run away if you don't like somebody's reaction.

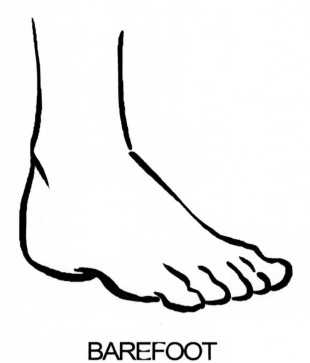

BAREFOOT

Remember: Go Barefoot At Home

Must I Adopt A Barefoot Lifestyle?

Must I adopt a barefoot lifestyle?

Remember the *Seinfeld* episode in which Jerry turns down the chance for a ménage à trois because he doesn't want to become an "orgy guy?" He worries that joining a three-some would force him to grow a mustache, get shag carpeting and change his friends.

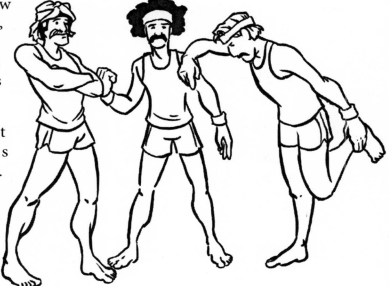

Barefoot running is *not* like that. You can run barefoot without changing your entire life.

Will I burn more calories running barefoot?

On any given run, it's hard to say. You may run more efficiently, thereby burning fewer calories. On the other hand, when you seem to flow rather than pound, you may run faster or farther, using more total energy.

The goal of barefoot running is to enable a lifetime of healthy running. Years of exercising rather than being injured and couch-bound will lead to many more calories burned.

Will my bare feet attract hot guys/gals?

Running with bare feet is bound to stimulate conversation. Where you take that conversation is up to you.

Can I wear a hat while I run barefoot?

Yes. Running barefoot need not be a political statement about minimalism or nudity or anything like that. Barefoot runners go without shoes because it's the most functional and enjoyable choice. Other clothing and equipment choices are entirely up to you.

On a cold day, your feet will lose more heat than they would in shoes and socks. In winter, I usually run wearing gloves and a hat. Sometimes this amuses passersby.

Is there a club for this in my area?

Possibly. Interest in barefoot running is growing, and you may be able to find a club on meetup.com or on Facebook. While it's always fun to share an experience with kindred spirits, you don't need a club to run barefoot.

Internet resources on barefoot running include:

- RunBarefootRunHealthy.com,
- BarefootRunners.org, the Barefoot Runners Society,
- Barefoot Ken Bob's website, barefootkenbob.com, and
- *Runner's World* barefoot running forums at tinyurl.com/rwbarefoot.

What about diet? I'm not vegetarian or anything like that.

It's not required. Even barefoot, I enjoy bacon as much as ever.

Would wearing socks ruin the benefits of barefoot running?

Socks will slightly reduce ground feedback, but not as much as shoes do. Unfortunately, socks don't last very long, and on certain surfaces, socks might snag and trip you up, or increase the chances of slipping.

Some runners have experimented with socks (for the cold) dipped in "Plasti Dip."

I like having pretty feet. I'm afraid this will ruin my feet.

Aboriginal people, who have never worn shoes, have wide feet with splayed toes. It's not dainty, but it *is* extremely healthy and functional. Some would say that strong and healthy is attractive.

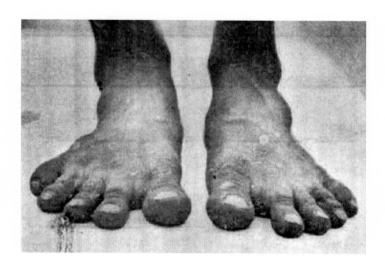

At the other extreme, we have foot binding, practiced for centuries among the well to do in China. Intended to give women small and "attractive" lotus shaped feet, this practice left women crippled and in pain for life.

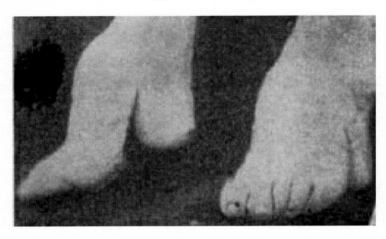

Only you can decide where on the form-function continuum you would rather be.

While a barefoot runner may have a wide forefoot and a somewhat thicker sole, the feet themselves, lacking corns, bunions, blisters, blackened toenails, and smell, are generally more attractive than habitually shod feet.

On the topic of pretty feet, be sure to read the interview with Heather Wiatrowski.

Can I play other sports barefoot? Basketball? Soccer? Tennis?

In many team sports, the danger is that shod teammates will step on your feet. I wouldn't participate barefoot in a sport where the other athletes wore studded or spiked shoes.

I spoke to one tennis player who grew up playing barefoot on hard courts in the Florida sun. When we give them the chance, our feet are extremely strong and adaptable.

What about outside the U.S.? Do people run barefoot elsewhere?

Walking and running barefoot seems relatively common all around the world. Some cities have "barefoot walking paths" especially cleared to encourage people to take off their shoes.

While stationed in Japan, US Marine Brad Kilpatrick ran his 23 miles of an ekiden [24 hour relay race] barefoot, after losing one of his shoes at the start. He had no previous barefoot running experience, and suffered no injuries from this unforeseen experiment.

A world-traveling friend reports yet another military-themed barefoot sighting:

> "I first saw someone running barefoot (other than on a beach) when I saw a pack of young army recruits running barefoot through sub-urban Cairo – a place where you don't want to be barefoot."

Any good anecdotes about barefoot running?

A few months ago, my corporate lawyer friend Sarah was inspired to go for a barefoot run in Palo Alto, in the wealthy heart of Silicon Valley. During her run, a woman pulled up beside her in a minivan and asked "in a very kind voice" whether Sarah needed a ride somewhere.

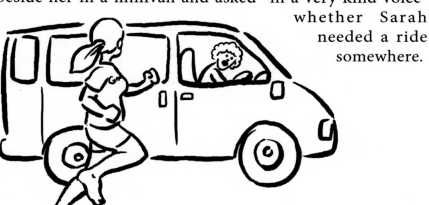

What is the best response to people who stare at my bare feet, or comment about it?

Smile. People who yell out to a barefoot runner are trying to make a connection. Your reaction sets the tone of the interaction. When you are positive, it plants the seed, "Hey, that barefoot runner was pretty cool. Maybe there's something to this barefoot running thing."

Remember, your exotic barefoot presence has made their day – given them something to go home and tell the kids about.

I will admit, when someone points out my bare feet, it makes me want to look down in mock horror and yell: "I've been mugged! Call the police!"

[**Summary:**   Barefoot running fits all lifestyles.]

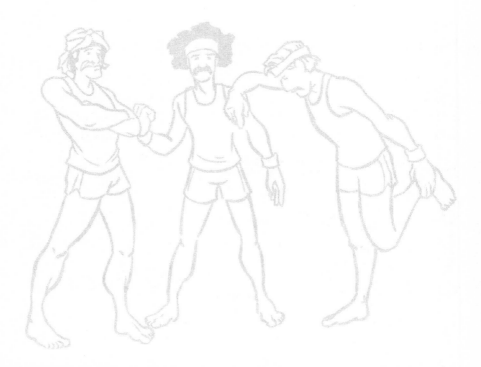

Interview:

Owen McCall: "Instead Of Thinking I'm Crazy, People Think I'm Some Sort Of Prophet"

And you are ...?

Owen McCall. I'm 57, and I live in Highland Park, Illinois, just 30 miles north of Chicago. I recently retired from doing molecular biology research for a large pharmaceutical company.

How did you start running?

Owen: My wife and I were fanatic bikers until the kids came along. Then you can't take all day off and bike for 100 miles. So I said, "What can I do when the kids are asleep?" And that was running. Like almost everybody else who runs, I found I was injured at least once or twice a year – injured to the degree that I couldn't run for weeks at a stretch. And I did that for about 15 years.

I had a typical runner's career. I ran a marathon, and was injured at the starting line ... but I finished it. I felt like I'd been mugged afterwards.

I continued that very typical story of runners – dreading that next injury and searching the *Runner's World* shoe issue for the perfect shoe that would solve all my biomechanical problems that were causing me to be injured.

Then my sister, a physical therapist in Dallas, traveled around the world and wrote this book [*The McCall Body Balance Method*] about natural movement in pre-industrial societies. So I looked at pictures of naked Greek fishermen pulling nets on the beach, and women carrying pots on their heads through the savanna or whatever, and I was intrigued by this idea that people who don't sit by the computer all day, who actually move all day, seem to do everything differently than we do.

Unfortunately, she didn't have a chapter in there on running. So, I thought, "Heck, I'll just go out there and run like those people walk. Just has to be right to do it barefoot."

So you came up with this yourself?

Owen: Yes, this was my own crazy idea. To avoid getting injured, you've got to get rid of what's been causing it, which must be the shoes, because people don't have these problems when they don't wear shoes.

So I immediately ran out, and got a stress fracture.

This was 10 years ago. That put me in the pool, swimming for six weeks. Then, I went out and did it again. Then, I went out and did it a third time. So, in my first year of barefoot running, I had three stress fractures.

Being kind of thick headed, I thought only after the third incident, "Maybe I'm doing this wrong. I wonder if anybody else has figured this out." That's when I stumbled onto Barefoot Ken Bob. I went to his site, and started e-mailing him. He told me that what I'd been doing wrong was going from one extreme form of running to the other. When you're running in trainers with those big heels, you're throwing out your heels in front of you, and you're heel striking. When you start running barefoot, you can't heel strike because it just hurts too much. So instead of running on my heels, I felt I needed to run on my forefoot. I was running like a sprinter.

I was pushing off, and I was running so my heel would hardly even touch the ground. Also, I was a pretty high-mileage runner, so I immediately shifted from 20 or 30 miles a week in trainers to 20 or 30 miles a week barefoot. In hindsight, it's pretty obvious that's what caused those stress fractures.

Ken Bob taught me that you really don't want to heel strike or forefoot strike. You don't want to strike anything. You want to land mid-foot, distributing the weight between the forefoot and the heel. Bend your knees and use a very high cadence – take very short steps. You don't want to feel any shock – ever. As soon as I started doing that … well, that was nine years ago, and I haven't had an injury in nine years.

In your opinion, what's the number one reason to run barefoot?

Owen: To avoid injury.

What about the smell?

Owen: Bare feet don't smell. Back in the 19th century, there was an expression: "an odor like a motorman's glove." Nobody knows what that means anymore. People don't even know what a motorman is. But a motorman was a guy who drove trolleys, and as part of his uniform, he had to wear gloves, which he wore all day long. His hands would sweat all day, so his hands would stink.

Same thing with shoes. You wear shoes and socks, you wear them all day long, and your feet are going to smell like a motorman's glove. They will stink.

If you don't put on shoes and socks, your feet are out in the fresh air. You will not get any stink in your feet – just as your hands won't stink if you're not wearing gloves.

Any favorite running anecdotes?

Owen: I was running my usual run, a couple of blocks from my house, and I had to cross a railroad track (next to the railroad station). I run this way a couple of hundred times a year, and for some reason, a policeman happened to be there. He saw me, and I noticed this look come over his face. He came running over, yelling, "Sir, sir! Stop, stop!"

What's the problem, I wonder, what could I possibly have been doing wrong? He tells me – "look me in the eye, look me in the eye!" and I'm looking him in the eye. And he sort of stops talking and this chagrined look comes over his face, and he says, "I'm sorry, you know, I just had this image in my mind that you have escaped from the mental hospital." He thought because I was running barefoot, I must be a lunatic who climbed down a bed sheet at the county insane asylum and was hotfooting it away.

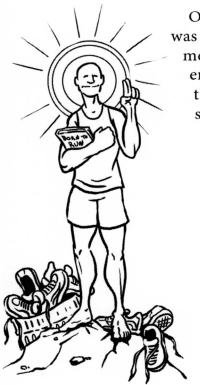

Of course, this was before *Born to Run* was published. That's the book that turned me from a lunatic into a luminary. Everything has changed. Now, instead of thinking I'm crazy, people think I'm some kind of prophet.

Will I Injure Myself Running Barefoot?

Will I injure myself running barefoot?

Yes, you will.

What? There must be a misunderstanding. If I go barefoot and do everything you say, won't I run injury-free forever after? Isn't that the whole point? Give me my money back!

Look. A large proportion of runners suffer injuries – with estimates as high as 75% each year. If you run, barefoot or not, you will inevitably end up with some soreness or other injury. Anecdotal and scientific evidence strongly suggest that barefoot running is healthier than running shod, but bare feet are not a cloak of invincibility.

You will have fewer injuries running barefoot than you would have running shod, but you will almost certainly suffer minor aches and pains, and occasionally something more severe.

Since going barefoot offers the likelihood of running into your sixties and beyond, you'll still be stubbing your toes and stepping on acorns at an age when many of your high school classmates spend their days getting fat in their La-Z-Boy recliners. Is that worth it to you?

What's the most serious injury report you've heard from a barefoot runner?

You know those spike strips outside parking lots that are labeled "WARNING! DO NOT BACK UP!! SEVERE TIRE DAMAGE!!!"

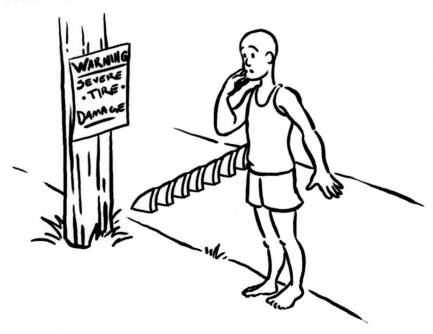

Wandering around in a crowd before the Santa Monica 10K, 36-year-old barefoot runner Burt Malcuit ignored the big warning signs, and walked right into one of those strips. The strip ripped up Burt's foot, and if his physician parents had been anywhere around, they would have sent him straight to the ER for stitches, and then to bed.

Fortunately, his dad wasn't there, so our hero decided to run, open wound and all. He didn't bleed to death, and he finished the race.

By this point, it was too late to get stitches, and in Burt's own words, "This is gonna take awhile to heal as it looks like someone tried to amputate my toe with a hand saw." So after taking 12 days off to let his foot mend, Burt followed up the injury with a 61-mile week – at that point his highest mileage ever.

I asked Burt whether he considered going out and just buying a pair of running shoes after all this.

Burt: "It never crossed my mind."

Indeed, even if I (your author) were to take a month off after stepping on a spike strip, my average weekly mileage for the year would still be ahead of my shod mileage in past years.

What are all the tradeoffs I need to consider?

As I've said, many injured runners find that their shin splints, IT Band Syndrome, plantar fasciitis and other chronic injuries disappear when they start running barefoot.

In exchange for this lack of injury, there are some tradeoffs. I'll summarize the main ones (again):

- ▸ When running barefoot, you will inevitably step on stones and acorns that will make you go "Ouch."
- ▸ Occasionally you will stub a toe, and it will hurt.
- ▸ Occasionally, you will get a splinter.
- ▸ Running in extremes of hot and cold, at night and on rocky trails, is more difficult when barefoot. Especially in the beginning, you may need to limit when and where you run.
- ▸ Your feet will get dirty.

You mention splinters. How do you remove them?

Splinters tend to work themselves out in a day or two. They are a minor inconvenience, and in my experience, very rare.

You mention stubbing your toe. That hurts! Can I break a toe?

A stubbed toe is probably the most frequent barefoot running injury. I've learned to look where I run, and I've also found that my feet have grown stronger over time, so when I stub my toes (at home, on a chair) nowadays, they no longer hurt.

I've never broken a toe, even when stubbed on a broken sidewalk with all my weight behind it. In fact, it was after I stubbed my toe for the first time, and noticed the next day that I felt my injury most when wearing shoes, and not at all when barefoot, that I really became a believer.

Won't competitors step on my feet in huge races like the New York City Marathon?

In the middle of the pack, there's not that much contact between runners.

I'd hesitate to run barefoot in a race where the other competitors were wearing spikes. But in road races, it's not an issue.

Is there significantly increased wear and tear on the knees and shins while running barefoot?

Both scientific and anecdotal evidence suggest that barefoot running results in less impact on the legs. [PAPER2] [PAPER8]

Shoes don't reduce your body weight or the force of your body moving toward the ground. They reduce the perception of impact. By dulling the pain you would otherwise feel, they allow you to really beat yourself up and do long-term damage.

How do you keep from acquiring diseases, tiny worms and other items that shoes protect you from?

These may be a problem in some tropical climates, but very rarely in the continental U.S. – certainly not enough to outweigh the benefits of going barefoot.

This question illustrates a very general social phenomenon exacerbated by TV news: disproportionate fear of very rare events. It's similar to the fear of plane crashes that leads people to drive long distances rather than fly, although the data clearly show that driving is many, many times more dangerous than air travel.

Yes, if you decide to run barefoot, freaky bad things could conceivably happen. But most of the time, you'll be happier and better off for all of the reasons I've outlined.

How does running without cushioning affect my joints?

Running without shoes allows your feet to feel the ground, so that you naturally run with good form, reducing the force of impact with the ground, and the force felt by your joints. [VIDEO4]

Don't my feet need protection from the hard ground?

Your feet are an important sensory organ. Being able to feel the ground allows you to smoothly and safely move your body through space. Imagine trying to walk or run if you could not feel the ground at all.

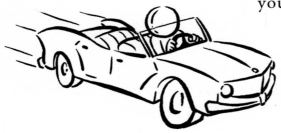

You no more want to protect your feet by cutting off sensory input than you would protect your head by cutting off its sensory inputs with a giant rubber-ball helmet.

How many times have you found a nail in your car tire, and you have no idea where you ran over it? What makes you think your feet won't suffer the same fate?

First of all, these doomsday scenarios don't occur very often. And when they do, you will recover, as we heard from Burt Malcuit.

And yes, part of running barefoot is choosing not to run through construction zones, and part of it is watching for hazards on the path ahead of you – though not looking straight down at your feet.

Whenever I see a nail or other metal debris in the road, I pick it up and carry it with me to the nearest trash can. Please join me in keeping our environment clean and safe for runners and bikers.

I know of at least two people who got stress fractures after they started barefoot.

So do I. But they weren't running barefoot (skin to ground). Both of them were pretend barefoot running – in minimalist shoes.

Okay, if you read the interview with Owen McCall, you know that barefoot runners can get a stress fracture. And you also know that it is extremely unlikely, especially if you follow the suggestions on good running form.

Will I bleed?

Although cuts to the foot are rare, they can happen when running barefoot or in shoes. If you have a medical condition like hemophilia, please check with your doctor before going on a barefoot run.

What about athlete's foot?

Athlete's foot is a fungal infection of the skin, and seems to thrive in a moist environment. What could be more moist than the inside of your shoe when you are exercising?

What else do you do for injury prevention?

Besides stretching, not much is necessary. I choose where I run, avoiding construction zones and rocky trails, and that's about it.

To once again quote Dr. Hoffman, "It is very significant that in the one hundred eighty six pairs of (bare) primitive feet examined, I did not find a single foot associated with the symptoms of weakness so characteristic and common in adult shoe-wearing feet, which are weakened by the restraint the shoe exerts over function." [PAPER14, p. 20]

What happens if you get injured? Is it okay to use cushioned shoes to protect your feet, or is it better not to run at all while recovering?

Only you can judge your particular situation, but I find rest to be the best recovery. Many runners find aqua-jogging in a pool to be a good short-term substitute.

If I start running barefoot, and it doesn't appear to go well, what warning signs should I look out for?

Running and walking barefoot has worked for humans since pre-historic times, so it should work for you too.

The most common problems are:

- ► *Top of foot pain* may be caused by doing too much, too soon, while barefoot.

  - ✚ Take it as slowly as your body needs, particularly if you are used to wearing shoes at home.

- ► *Blisters* are a sure sign of pushing off with the feet while barefoot.

  - ✚ Remember to "lift" your feet without pushing.

- ► Many injuries may result from running "barefoot" in minimalist shoes without first having learned good form. Light shoes make it easy to push too hard.

  - ✚ Feedback from sensitive bare soles helps rein in our tendency to overdo it. Go bare.

Summary: Bare feet are not a cloak of invincibility. But they're a big step in the right direction.

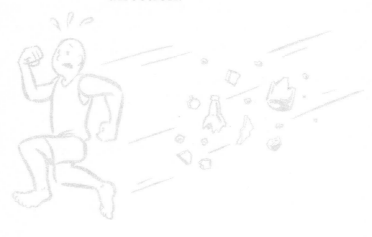

Interview:

Efrem Rensi: "If There's Ever Been A Time For Barefoot Running ... It's Now"

And you are ... ?

Efrem Rensi. I'm 38, and I'm a graduate student in mathematics at the University of California at Davis.

Why do you think barefoot running is so popular nowadays?

Efrem: I think it's a very modern thing. I really think paved roads are what made barefoot running accessible to all – as recreation. Most natural surfaces are a mixed bag – some are runner-friendly, and some are not. Frankly, I don't know what a natural surface is, because there are very few entirely natural surfaces.

Right, it's not a golf course.

Efrem: What people typically consider a natural surface – a trail or a hill with gravel – is quite uncomfortable. Barefoot running is made much more pleasant by having clean, smooth streets in a relatively clean environment.

What led you to barefoot running?

Efrem: When I was 31, I rode my bicycle around a lot, and I hurt my knee riding my bike. I thought, "I'll take up running." But when I tried to run, my knee hurt.

I went to see the doctor about my knee injury, and the doctor told me that I overpronate, and that I was exacerbating this injury just by walking around all day.

He recommended that I go to a store in Berkeley that had specialty running shoes. They looked at me and said, "Okay, you overpronate. You need a motion-control shoe."

I was fascinated by this whole thing. Whenever I have an injury, I research it intensively. I started looking at the Internet, at different kinds of shoes. I wanted to see what kind of shoe would be best for me. After several months, I ended up finding Barefoot Ken Bob's [barefoot running] website. It really struck a chord with me.

How did you transition?

Efrem: At first, I had a lot of problems. My ankle hurt a lot, and I thought, "Maybe barefoot running isn't for me." I didn't start running again until I'd been walking barefoot for several months. I was just going for walks barefoot and going for hikes barefoot. My ultimate goal was to start running barefoot. The first run I did was for 17 minutes.

Now your marathon PR is 3:15. You've come a long way!

Efrem: I would say I belong to the league of very low-level competitive runners.

Why do you think barefoot running is better than running in shoes? Performance?

Efrem: I enjoy it more. I feel like I'm doing something that's not selfish. Barefoot running is bigger than me. It's a whole different way of experiencing the world. It's more interesting. Running in shoes was never that interesting to me. I did it because I wanted to lose some weight or something. Now, I actually enjoy the running.

Don't your feet get dirty?

Efrem: Yes, my feet get dirty. Afterwards, I go home, and take a shower. I use one of those little green and yellow 3M scrub sponges.

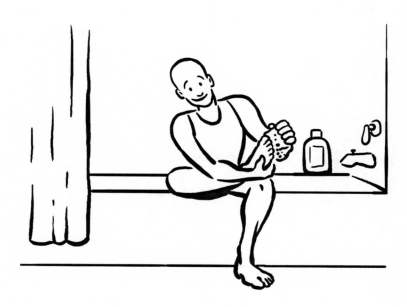

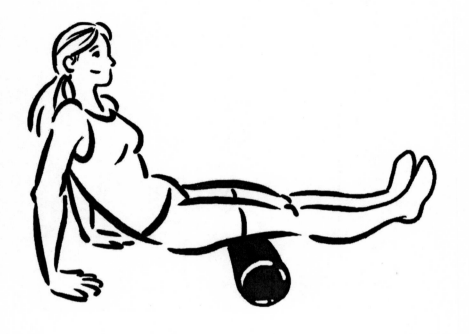

Remember: Roll That Foam Roller!

Environmental Impact

What is the environmental impact of running shoes?

The carbon footprint of a single pair of 12oz running shoes is about 143 pounds of CO_2.

The soles are primarily made of rubber. The upper part of the shoe is made of some combination of nylon, polyester, thermoplastic urethane (TPA) and perhaps some breathable material. The mid-sole is made primarily of polyurethane or lighter ethylene vinyl acetate (EVA), which lasts up to 1,000 years in a landfill.

What about biodegradable shoes?

Why? Why even discuss how to make a biodegradable version of a product which is expensive, wasteful, very possibly injurious, and as you've been reading ... unnecessary?

But to answer your question: Brooks recently introduced a line of $140 "biodegradable" shoes, which they claim will decompose within 20 years in a landfill.

Brooks has another line of shoes made from recycled CDs and old sofas. No word on whether you can have a shoe custom-made from a collection of your favorite albums – the soundtrack to *Chariots of Fire*, say.

If I decide to go barefoot, can I recycle my old shoes?

Yes. Shoe manufacturers have programs to recycle your shoes for materials. This is one case where I prefer to recycle than to reuse.

Where are these shoes made, anyway?

These days, most running shoes are made in China and Southeast Asia by contract manufacturers. Typically, the factories are not owned by the U.S. companies that brand and market the shoes to us.

New Balance still makes a small proportion of its shoes in North America, but the trend is to move overseas, where costs are lower, and labor laws are less stringent.

It's hard to measure the impact of the manufacturing process on the health of the workers. Consumers International reports that many workers are ill-treated and ill-paid, with just 0.4% of the retail price of a running shoe going to worker's salaries.

How long do running shoes last?

According to a *Runner's World* survey, the average runner buys 3.1 pairs of running shoes per year. In other words, the average pair of running shoes lasts a little under four months. That's a lot of cash out of your pocket, and a lot of shoes in landfills.

I recently saw a pair of Nike Mayfly shoes labeled "Engineered to last for 100km of running." 100 kilometers (about 62 miles) is less than many competitive runners log in a single week. Imagine the waste, not to mention the expense, of buying a new pair of shoes each week!

What's the future of running shoes?

We've already discussed "minimalist" running shoes, which claim to allow "barefoot style running," while still giving big shoe companies something to sell.

Beyond minimalism, "green" running shoes are all the rage, reports *The New York Times*, and each shoe manufacturer has its own angle – vegan shoes, recyclable shoes, Fair Trade shoes, eco-friendly sustainable shoes … you name it, you can buy it.

All the major shoe companies, whether driven by principle or external pressure, are doing a much better job of using green materials and processes, providing transparency into their supply chains, eliminating child labor, etc., than they did a decade ago.

But at the end of the day, a shoe company exists to sell shoes. Their designers or their marketing people might look at the research referenced in this book, but even at their environmental best, they are never going to come out and say, "You know what, Mr. and Mrs. Jones? You and your kids would really be so much better off without shoes."

So, what's the green angle on something completely unnecessary? Eliminate it. Send green running shoes the way of the shoe-fitting x-ray. We can do it.

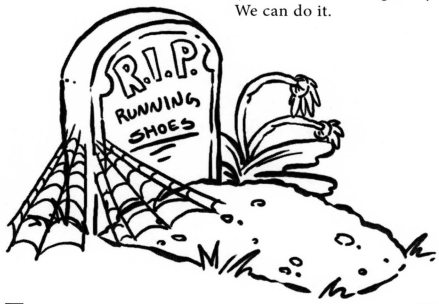

Summary: Going barefoot is a great way to reduce your footprint on the earth.

Just The Facts

10 Reminders – Copy And Review

Go barefoot at home

Lift your feet

Bend your knees

Don't push off

Stand tall

Relax

Keep your hips forward

Take quick light steps

Keep a neutral neck

Roll that foam roller!

Scientific Papers

PAPER1

Warburton M, Barefoot Running, SPORTSCIENCE, 2001

- ▶ In brief: fewer injuries, more efficient.
- ▶ Full text: http://tinyurl.com/firstpaper

PAPER2

Burkett LN, Kohrt WM, Buchbinder R., Effects of shoes and foot orthotics on VO2 and selected frontal plane knee kinematics, *Med Sci Sports Exerc. 1985 Feb;17(1):158-63.*

- ▶ In brief: mass of shoes (and orthotics) slows you down and increases angular knee motion.
- ▶ Abstract: http://tinyurl.com/anchorsonyour-feet

PAPER3

Stewart SF, Footgear – its history, uses and abuses, *Clin Orthop Relat Res. 1972;88:119-30.*

- ▶ And I quote "…all writers who have reported their observations of barefoot peoples agree that the untrammeled feet of natural men are free from the disabilities commonly noted among shod people - hallux valgus, bunions, hammer toe and painful feet."
- ▶ Link: http://tinyurl.com/barefeetalwayshealthier

PAPER4

Lieberman DE, Venkadesan M, Werbel WA, Daoud AI, D'Andrea S, Davis IS, Mang'eni RO, Pitsiladis Y., Foot strike patterns and collision forces in habitually barefoot versus shod runners, Nature. 2010 Jan 28;463(7280):433-4.

- ► In brief: barefoot running reduces impact.
- ► Abstract: http://tinyurl.com/barefootnature

PAPER5

GR Clinghan, GP Arnold, TS Drew, LA Cochrane, RJ Abboud, Do you get value for money when you buy an expensive pair of running shoes, Br J Sports Med 2008;42:189-193 doi:10.1136/bjsm.2007.038844

- ► In brief: inexpensive shoes cushion as well as expensive running shoes. Maybe better.
- ► Abstract: http://tinyurl.com/cheaperbetter

PAPER6

Vormittag K, Calonje R, Briner WW., Foot and Ankle Injuries in the Barefoot Sports, Curr Sports Med Rep. 2009 Sep-Oct;8(5):262-6.

- ► In brief: shoes limit the feet's natural movement, and cause injury.
- ► Abstract: http://tinyurl.com/lowbarefootinjuryrate

PAPER7

Wells, LH: The Bantu Foot, American Journal of Physical Anthropology, Volume 15 Issue 2, pp 185-289, Jan/Mar1931

- ► In brief: the foot of the South African native ... was much healthier.
- ► Abstract: http://tinyurl.com/bantufoot

PAPER8

Divert C, Mornieux G, Baur H, Mayer F, Belli A., Mechanical comparison of barefoot and shod running, Int J Sports Med. 2005 Sep;26(7):593-8.

- ▶ In brief: bare feet experience *less* peak force.
- ▶ Abstract: http://tinyurl.com/lowerimpact

PAPER9

Richards CE, Magin PJ, Callister R., Is your prescription of distance running shoes evidence-based?

- ▶ In brief: there is no scientific evidence to recommend cushioned arch-supported, heel-raised running shoes.
- ▶ Abstract: http://tinyurl.com/noevidencefor-shoes

PAPER10

Divert C, Mornieux G, Freychat P, Baly L, Mayer F, Belli A., Barefoot-shod running differences: shoe or mass effect?, Int J Sports Med. 2008 Jun;29(6):512-8. Epub 2007 Nov 16.

- ▶ In brief: why do shod runners use more oxygen?
- ▶ Abstract: http://tinyurl.com/shoeormass

PAPER11

B. Zipfel, L.R. Berger, Shod versus unshod: The emergence of forefoot pathology in modern humans, The Foot, Volume 17, Issue 4, Pages 205-213 (December 2007)

- ▶ In brief: the more we wear shoes, the unhealthier our feet are.
- ▶ Abstract: http://tinyurl.com/shoescausepathology

PAPER12

Kerrigan DC, Franz JF, Keenan GS, Dicharry J, Della Croce U, Wilder RP, The Effect of Running Shoes on Lower Extremity Joint Torques, PM&R Volume 1, Issue 12 , Pages 1058-1063, December 2009

- ► In brief: running shoes may damage our knees, hips and ankles.
- ► Abstract: http://tinyurl.com/shoesmaydamage

PAPER13

Trinkaus, Erik: Anatomical evidence for the antiquity of human footwear use. 2005 Journal of Archaeological Science 32(10):1515-1526.

- ► In brief: when we wear shoes, we use our toes less, so they wither away.
- ► Overview: http://tinyurl.com/toesatrophyinshoes

PAPER14

Hoffman, Phil. 1905, Conclusions Drawn from a Comparative Study of Barefoot and Shoe-Wearing Peoples, The Journal of Bone and Joint Surgery, 1905;s2-3:105-136

- ► In brief: shoes "deform" and "cripple" the feet.
- ► Full text: http://tinyurl.com/footcompare

PAPER15

Oleson T, Flocco W. Randomized controlled study of premenstrual symptoms treated with ear, hand, and foot reflexology. Obstet Gynecol 1993;82:906-911.

- ▸ In brief: reflexology reduces symptoms of PMS.
- ▸ Abstract (see sidebar): http://tinyurl.com/reflexologystudy

PAPER16

2008 NIH Glucosamine/chondroitin Arthritis Intervention Trial Primary Study

- ▸ In brief: "For a subset of participants with moderate-to-severe pain, glucosamine combined with chondroitin sulfate provided statistically significant pain relief compared with placebo."
- ▸ Overview: http://tinyurl.com/gluco4knees

PAPER17

Csapo, R., Maganaris, C. N., Seynnes, O. R. and Narici, M. V. (2010). On muscle, tendon and high heels. J. Exp. Biol. 213, 2582-2588.

- ▸ In brief: wearing high heels leads to shorter muscles and thicker, stiffer Achilles tendons.
- ▸ Overview: http://tinyurl.com/notoheels

Articles

ARTICLE1

Why Shoes Make "Normal" Gait Impossible.

- ▶ by William A Rossi, D.P.M.
- ▶ http://tinyurl.com/abnormalgait

ARTICLE2

Barefoot Running: A Natural Step For The Endurance Athlete?

- ▶ by Dennis G. Driscoll, Head XC Coach, Natick (MA) High School.
- ▶ http://tinyurl.com/coachingbarefoot

ARTICLE3

Orthopedic surgeon Joseph Froncioni discusses shoes. Read about his call to Nike!

- ▶ http://tinyurl.com/surgeonsays

ARTICLE4

Home page for the biomechanics lab of Prof. Daniel E. Lieberman at Harvard University.

- ▶ http://tinyurl.com/liebermanlab

ARTICLE5

The Myth of Running Shoe Cushioning

- ► Running shoes do not reduce and may even increase impact felt by runners.
- ► http://tinyurl.com/cushioningmyth

ARTICLE6

U.S. Army says matching shoes to foot type is "sports myth."

- ► http://tinyurl.com/sportsmyth

ARTICLE7

"No consumer could reasonably be misled into thinking vitaminwater was a healthy beverage."

- ► http://tinyurl.com/donotdrinkthis

Books

BOOK1

Take Off Your Shoes and Walk : Steps to Better Foot Health

- ► By Simon J. Wikler D.S.C. (1961)
- ► A foot doctor describes the source and history of foot problems.
- ► See an extract of the book at http://tinyurl.com/takeoffyourshoes

BOOK2

Foot Troubles

- ► By Bernarr MacFadden (1926)
- ► An investigation of feet by an eccentric yet very insightful thinker.
- ► http://tinyurl.com/foottroubles

BOOK3

Born to Run

- ► By Christopher McDougall (2009)
- ► This is the book that brought barefoot running to the attention of 21st century America. A terrifically readable story.

Videos

VIDEO1

Sammy Wanjiru wins the 2008 Olympic Marathon – watch his bent knees and effortless form!

- ► http://tinyurl.com/bentknees
- ► (As we go to print, this video has been removed from youtube "on copyright grounds." Let's hope it is reinstated. Wanjiru's running form was a thing of beauty.)

VIDEO2

Side by side video from Dr. Marc Silberman at the NJ Sports Medicine Clinic. Watch how shoes force a runner to heel strike. A must see!

- ► http://tinyurl.com/seebothtogether

VIDEO3

Julian Romero relaxed after the 2010 Chicago Marathon:

- ► http://tinyurl.com/julianrunschicago

VIDEO4

From the leading scientific journal Nature, featuring Harvard professor Daniel Lieberman. See for yourself the graph of impact forces on the legs:

- ► http://tinyurl.com/naturevideo

VIDEO5

Terry Fox run – not barefoot, but absolutely inspiring:

- ► http://tinyurl.com/runacrosscanada

VIDEO6

Dejen Gebremeskel wins an elite race on one shoe. Why are the commentators so very convinced that the "hard track" will hurt him?

- ► http://tinyurl.com/oneshoe

Exercises For The Barefoot Runner

Much of the standard running exercise regimen involves strengthening the body to withstand the pounding of running. Barefoot running reduces impact, thereby reducing the need for all that strengthening. That said, running in a straight line on flat surfaces for long distances creates imbalances that will compound the natural asymmetry of our bodies.

The following are some excellent exercises to strengthen common weak points for all runners – the quads/thighs and the hips. The possible menu of exercises is infinite, so feel free to customize a routine to meet your own body's needs.

While I don't go to *Runner's World* for shoe advice, their recommendations on strengthening, stretching, and diet, are useful and readable. Just avert your eyes from the ads.

Wall Sits (strengthens quads/thighs to combat runner's knee)

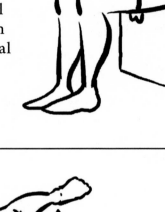

- ▶ Sit against a wall as shown, with your legs out at a 90 degree angle in front of you.

- ▶ You will feel this in your quads/thighs.

- ▶ Hold for as long as you can, take a rest, and repeat.

- ▶ Over time, your legs will strengthen till you can hold this pose for several minutes.

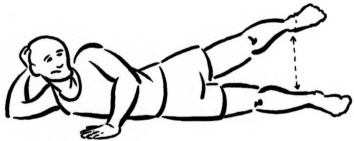

Side Leg Raise (strengthens hips, combats IT Band Syndrome)

- ▶ Lie on left side, relaxed, with legs straight out, ankle bent.

- ▶ Raise and lower right leg, 20-30x.

- ▶ Repeat lying on right side.

- ▶ Work up to 3 sets of 30 repetitions per side.

One-Legged Stands And Squats (strengthen muscles around knee – more advanced than wall sits)

- A fun exercise to do anywhere!
- Stand on one leg.
- Bend the knee of your weighted leg to lower and raise yourself.
- Vary how low you go.
- Vary the position of the free leg – straight out in front of you, behind you, and to the side.
- See how long you can stand on one leg.
- Eventually, you may graduate to doing this on an unstable surface, such as a BOSU.
- Running is a succession of transitions from one-legged stands. If you aren't stable on one foot, how will you be stable running?

Clam Shell (strengthen glutes)

- Lie on one side, knees bent at 90 degrees.
- Lift your top leg, hinging at the hip and ankle, 20x.

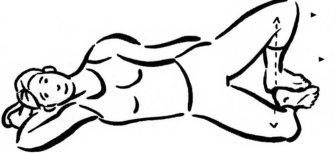

- Repeat on other side.
- Work up to 3 sets of 30 per side.

Front Lunge (strengthen quads)

- Do not do this if you suffer from knee instability. Work up to lunges by doing wall sits and one-legged stands for as many months as it takes to strengthen your quads and stabilize your knee.

- Start standing straight, with feet hip width and toes pointing forward.

- Take a big step forward with your right foot so that your right thigh is parallel to the floor and your right knee is above your forefoot – no further forward than your toes.

- Left leg is bent, with only the ball of your back foot on the ground.

- Keep a wide enough stance so you don't topple sideways.

- Keep your torso erect.

- Push upward with your right leg to return to a standing position. (Or if you have the space to do a "walking lunge," continue forward with the other leg.)

- Repeat.

- Work up to 3 sets of 10 on each side.

Side Lunge (strengthen hips, glutes)

- Start with feet parallel and hip width apart
- Step to the right, keeping weight on heels and feet forward.
    - Keep shifting weight to the right, so that your knee drops forward over your right foot – not out to the side.
        - Keep your torso erect yet relaxed, and use your hands comfortably for balance.
            - Push with your leg to return to center.
                - Repeat – work up to 3 sets of 10 on each side.

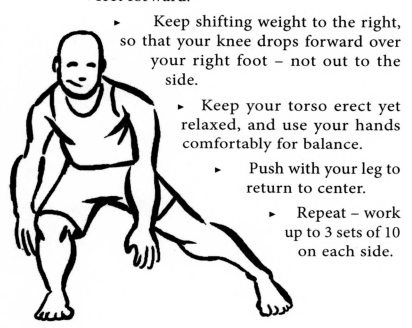

Donkey Kick (Strengthen hips, glutes)

- Get down on your hands and knees, with back parallel to the floor.
- Move one knee forward and back, as shown.
- Repeat.

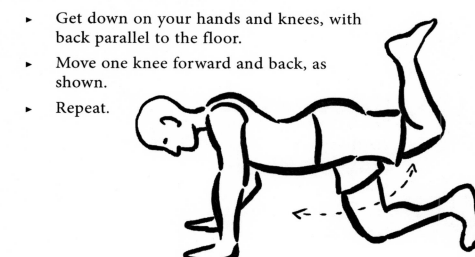

Ab Strengthening / Elbow Planks

- ▶ Hold your body in a straight line, with abs and butt tensed.

- ▶ Be sure not to let your butt stick up, nor to sag in the middle.

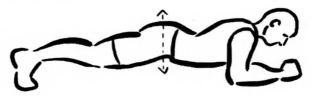

- ▶ Work up to 10 sets of 30 seconds each.

- ▶ Safer and better than sit ups.

Overhead Squat (ab reset)

- ▶ Begin in a wide stance with your toes pointed slightly out.

- ▶ Hold a light bar above your head – this is just to help you keep good form. With your elbows locked and your neck in a neutral position, your arms should be slightly behind your ears.

- ▶ Keeping your back very straight, shoulders pulled back:

- ▶ Send your hips back

- ▶ Bend your knees into the squat position.

- ▶ Straighten up to the starting position.

- ▶ Clench your glutes to finish.

- ▶ Do just a few of these before each run

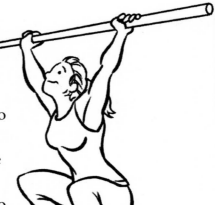

Stretching

Start your runs with a gentle warm up, either by walking or very slowly running for several minutes. Do not stretch cold muscles.

While running barefoot will reduce impact and impact-related injuries, you still need to watch out for muscle tightness and imbalances. The following stretches are great after you've finished your run and cool-down walk.

Piriformis aka Figure 4 Stretch (excellent for butt/glutes)

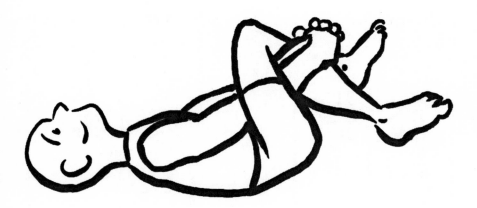

Sitting Piriformis Stretch

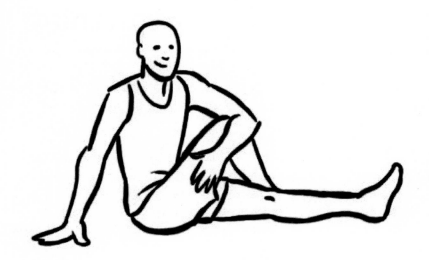

Calf Stretch – with back knee bent, and with back knee straight.

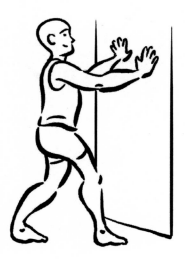 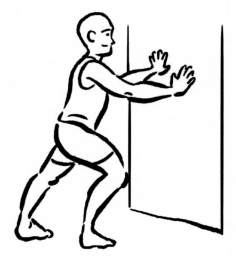

Quad/Thigh Stretch

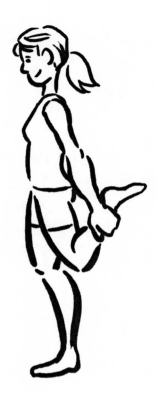

Hurdler Stretch (butt/glutes)

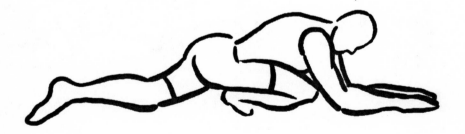

Roller stretches

The black (high density) foam roller is your friend. Buy one of these for $25 at a sporting goods store or on the Internet, and it will last you for years.

A few minutes on this twice a day can make all the difference for running injury free. I'm practically begging you – buy one of these, and use it regularly.

The more it hurts, especially on the side – the more you are tight and in danger of injury, and need this stretch. The pain will decrease over a few weeks of regular twice-daily use.

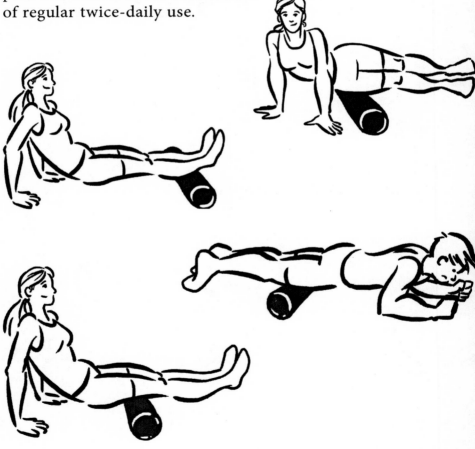

And once again: never run or exercise while on painkillers.

Other Resources For Athletes

RESOURCE1

Alexander Technique

I highly recommend Alexander Technique for athletes and musicians with tightness or injuries in or around the neck and back, or for anyone who wants to improve overall body mechanics.

To learn more, read *The Use of the Self*, or visit www.alexandertechnique.com.

RESOURCE2

Feldenkrais

1. openATM.org provides a variety of free Feldenkrais Awareness Through Movement lessons – like a much gentler version of yoga. Just amazing for reducing tension in the back and elsewhere. More lessons are available on iTunes, and on eBay.

2. The audio version of Dan Heggie's *Running With The Whole Body* is available on Amazon and elsewhere. Follow along as the author guides you through this sequence of movement lessons, relieving back tension while providing wonderful insight into the development of our ability to walk and run.

Epilogue

If you were moved to cast off your shoes and head out for a barefoot trot around the block, please email and let me know how it went. Likewise, if you have questions that remain unanswered, send them my way: ashish@runbare-footrunhealthy.com.

Many recent converts to barefoot running are so excited by their newfound health that they want all their friends to sign up. "How do I convince my friends to run barefoot?" is a common question.

My answer is, "Don't. Not one word." I tried for years to convince other runners with the facts, the analysis, and the miraculous personal anecdotes, and I came to realize that people will change their minds when they're ready, and not a moment sooner.

The best you can do is to keep running, stay healthy, and keep smiling. Inspire by example, not by nagging. (And consider giving this book as a birthday or Christmas present.) Then one day, when your friends show up for a run without their shoes, resist the urge to say, "I told you so!"

Speaking of inspiration, if this book inspired you, educated you, or made you question some of your assumptions, please help other runners by posting your review to Amazon.com.

Now get out there and run!

Lightning Source UK Ltd.
Milton Keynes UK
UKOW051418171011

180453UK00002B/3/P